Philosophy for nursing

Philosophy for nursing

Jan Reed RN, BA, PhD
Reader in Nursing
University of Northumbria at Newcastle
Newcastle upon Tyne, UK

Ian Ground BA
Development Officer for Liberal Adult Education
Newcastle University
Newcastle upon Tyne, UK

FOREWORD BY
Margaret Dunlop RN, BA, MEd, D Nur Sci
Professor of Nursing, Griffith University
Queensland, Australia

A member of the Hodder Headline Group
LONDON • SYDNEY • AUCKLAND

First published in Great Britain in 1997 by
Arnold, a member of the Hodder Headline Group
338 Euston Road, London NW1 3BH

Whilst the advice and information in this book is believed to be true and
accurate at the time of going to press, neither the author[s] nor the publisher
can accept any legal responsibility or liability for any errors or omissions
that may be made.

British Library Cataloguing in Publication Data
A catalogue record for this book is available from the British Library

Library of Congress Cataloging-in Publication Data
A catalog record for this book is available from the Library of Congress

ISBN 0 340 61028 X

Typeset in 10/12 pt Palatino by J&L Composition Ltd, Filey, North Yorkshire

Printed and bound in Great Britain by J.W. Arrowsmith Ltd, Bristol

Contents

Preface

In writing this book, we hoped to be able to do several things. Firstly, we hoped to provide nurses with an interest in the possibilities of philosophy with some form of overview of the subject, which would make its relevance to nursing clear and immediate. Having noticed the rise of references to philosophical work in nursing literature, we felt that this was an interest which was growing, but we also felt that without some background knowledge, many nurses reading this literature would not be able to critically evaluate the arguments made. The danger is that readers will either dismiss such references as pretentious, or be overimpressed by them. Authors who quote Plato or Heidegger or Wittgenstein may do this simply as a strategy for increasing their academic standing, in which case they should be challenged. Others, however, use these ideas as a way of stimulating debate or new ways of thinking about things. There is not much point in doing this, however, if their audience cannot participate. It seemed, therefore, that it would be useful to write some sort of guide which would help people to engage in what seems to be emerging as an important part of nursing debate.

The second aim that we hoped to achieve was to do some philosophy. The issues and problems facing nursing can, in some ways, be seen as very graphic and immediate examples of the sorts of problems that philosophy can address, and in a very useful way. The intriguing ambivalence of being people who are paid to care is one which is reflected in other areas of life, and other areas of philosophy, and so nursing can provide a rich and complex area for philosophy to work. Conversely, some of the debates in nursing seem amenable to philosophical inquiry, in the way that philosophy can provide a fresh way of looking at things.

The third, and perhaps most important aim that we wanted to achieve, was to kindle some enthusiasm for philosophy in nurses. As no one text can cover the range of philosophical writing, we hoped that the selected ideas that we discuss in this book would stimulate nurses to go and read more philosophy for themselves. This might happen because readers find philosophical ideas helpful and provide possible solutions or ways out of arguments, or it might happen because they find that they raise more questions, and it really does not matter which way it happens as long as it does.

With these different aims, the book has chapters which try to do different things. The first two chapters are about setting the scene. We cover the nature of philosophy, its history, methods and approaches, and discuss its relevance to nursing. Some readers may want to omit these chapters, particularly if they are familiar with these areas. From Chapter 3 to Chapter 8 we address some of the areas of philosophy which we see as being of particular relevance to nursing, giving an overview of the main positions, and looking at how these can be brought to bear on nursing problems. In the final chapter, we take a broader approach, looking at the move from task-centred to patient-centred nursing, and subjecting this change to philosophical analysis. The purpose of this chapter is not solely to address this issue, but also to show how a philosophical argument looks when it is laid out.

By having these chapters, with their different aims and forms, we think that we will have gone some way to achieving our aims, providing an overview of philosophy, doing philosophy, and interesting readers in philosophy.

Because this book (and most others in this book) mentions many writers and thinkers, but does not directly refer to specific works, we have decided to provide *references* only for those works directly referred to in the text. Our further reading lists will cover the other writers mentioned and give examples of particularly characteristic, important or accessible work, or discussions and summaries of this work. We will also give the details of books which cover areas generally, or which argue particular points which will be of interest. One problem in referencing books in philosophy is that there are often many editions of work by different publishers. We have tried to give the most recent editions in every case. When trying to find books, it is usually useful to search catalogues with the philosopher as author and as a subject, as many works have been translated, and will be listed under the translator's name.

Foreword

These are times of momentous change in nursing and in health care, both of which are in the process of being profoundly re-shaped. Some of the changes arise from within nursing itself as part of its professionalization project. Other changes are thrust upon nursing and nurses as governments struggle to contain health care while improving access, equity and health outcomes.

As old certainties lose their hold, new possibilities open up for redeveloping the place of nursing in health care. At the same time, new ethical issues are arising and political debates about the role of the state in health care and health-care provision continue.

In this climate of uncertainty and change, Jan Reed and Ian Ground have contributed this timely book which considers the interface of philosophy and nursing. Its content together with its lively, accessible style help clear space for the discussions and philosophical arguments we need to have as the ground shifts beneath our feet.

Similar to other oppressed groups, nursing has drawn selectively on philosophy to 'liberate' itself and to advance its professional projects (autonomy of practice, a body of knowledge and/or research agendas, for example). More rarely, nurses have used philosophy to critically evaluate nursing and its projects – to consider what should be its boundaries and limitations in the interests of society and those we claim to serve. Many of our truths, such as holistic care, seem self-evidently good and virtuous.

For those new to philosophy this book provides an excellent introduction, making visible the relevance of philosophical debate to nursing (and health-care) issues. They should, however, note the authors' repeated warnings that, in trying to give a very broad cover, they have inevitably simplified complex ideas and arguments. This book should be regarded as a way into the literature which is listed as further reading.

For those nurses more familiar with philosophical thought, the book opens up areas of potentially fruitful dialogue and argument. This I take to be the authors' intent – the opening up of questions and issues rather than their premature closure through information or ideology.

This book should not be taken as the final arbiter on links between philosophy and nursing but rather as suggestive of possible links in a way that opens them up for further exploration. It would be good to see further exploration of the issues raised in the last chapter, but there are other issues throughout the book, raised but not explored, that also merit further attention (for example, the theory–practice gaps). But the first essential for fruitful discussion and argument is the more philosophically literate nursing profession this book aims to create. For this I commend the authors and recommend the book.

Margaret Dunlop
Professor of Nursing
Griffith University
Queensland, Australia

Philosophy and nursing: an overview

Introduction

'Philosophy' is a word that is used in many different ways – to describe the obscure and impenetrable musings of long dead Ancients, to describe the casual speculations which occur when people have had too much to drink, or to describe the guidelines for practice pinned up in the office of hospital wards. In a sense, all of these uses are to some extent correct (with perhaps the exception of the drunk) if we take philosophy to mean a careful deliberation of ideas and issues. With this definition we all engage in philosophy at some time – the question is whether it is good philosophy or bad.

To produce good philosophy we need to return to the classical definition of the word, as attributed to Socrates, who described himself as a lover (*philos*) of wisdom (*sophia*). Using this definition we can start to ask about the nature of wisdom, and then ask if our thinking has moved us anywhere towards this goal. Wisdom, as one dictionary has it, is the ability to 'think and act utilising knowledge, experience, understanding, common sense, and insight'. Philosophy, then, is the pursuit of this, and wisdom is to be achieved by the careful thinking through and analysis of these things. It is important to note here the word 'act' which suggests that wisdom is of practical use, which leads to action, and it is not just a matter of contemplation. We should also note the inclusion of 'experience' as it indicates that wisdom is not purely abstract, and the words 'common sense', which we take to mean that wisdom does not consist of developing fanciful and high-flown ideas which are unintelligible to the rest of the world – there should be some common ground between the words of the wise and the ideas of the not so wise. The word 'insight' is a more difficult one as it is often used to describe mystical flashes of intuition, which, presumably cannot be acquired but simply waited for. Insight, however, can also be thought of as a corollary of understanding, which is something which can certainly be worked for.

This gives us some indication of what good philosophy should lead to, and therefore how it can be recognized. If our thinking leads us to more confusion, avoids difficult dilemmas, or is inconsistent, then this is not wisdom, and not good philosophy. If, however, as a result of our thinking, we find the questions more clearly defined, difficult areas tackled, and there is a coherence about our conclusions, then perhaps we have done some good philosophy.

Talking about philosophy in this way is, however, still very abstract, and certainly not enough to go very far on. What we hope to do in this book, therefore, is to show philosophy. We have taken a number of areas of philosophy which are of particular relevance to nursing and outlined the work that has been done in these areas. Remembering the action part of wisdom, we have also tried to show how this work can be brought to bear on problems and dilemmas which face nurses in practice. By discussing such real-life events, the usefulness of philosophy is, hopefully made clear. The book begins with this chapter, which is a brief discussion of philosophy and nursing, including an overview of the history of philosophy and the way that it has reflected and addressed the social issues of the time. The next chapter is devoted to a discussion of philosophical method, in other words how philosophical debates have been conducted, which includes a summary of logic. These two chapters will, we hope, prepare the reader for the rest of the book – although they are by no means compulsory they will help the reader to place the other chapters in some sort of philosophical context. In our final chapter, we lay out an analysis of contemporary issues in nursing, namely the change from task-orientated to patient-centred care, and in doing so hope to show how a philosophical discourse could be developed. We hope that it is good philosophy.

Knowledge in nursing – the limitations of research

In 1972, in the UK, a report was published, the Report of the Committee on Nursing, which later became known as the Briggs Report. Many UK nurses can quote one phrase from this report even if they know no other, and this phrase is 'Nursing should become a research-based profession'. This phrase was eagerly seized on by UK nurses as a call to research, and the development of academic nursing gained new momentum. The hope was that if nursing could develop a scientific knowledge base, then not only would patient care be improved, and outdated practices rejected, but nursing could develop a knowledge base which would mark it as distinct from other professions.

Nursing research, of course, did not start with the Briggs Report – historians of nursing often cite Florence Nightingale as an advocate of research and as inventor of the pie chart. Nor has nursing research been solely a UK activity. In the USA, Isabel Stewart was attempting to establish a research centre in the 1920s and in many other countries there have been efforts to promote nursing research to such an extent that Virginia Henderson (1982) reported that by 1967, when the first international conference on the nursing process was held, 'nursing science was in the ascendancy'.

Nursing science probably remains in the ascendancy today, but there are some indications that nursing is starting to explore more enthusiastically other forms of enquiry. These other forms of knowledge, for example, intuition, experiential learning and aesthetics, have always been a part of nursing knowledge, albeit less honoured than science, but they are beginning more and more to be the subject of formal academic debate. Some of these developments have arisen as people who teach nursing have embraced educational theories and have explored different ways of conveying to students the nature of nursing. This has involved the use of experiential learning theories, drama, poetry and visual art and is stimulated by ideas about reflective practice which do not conform to traditional ideas of rational science.

Carper (1978), in a seminal article, identified four types of nursing knowledge in practice, namely intuition, experience, aesthetics and ethics, and many others since have sought to understand these forms of knowledge. Patricia Benner, for example, looked at the knowledge that expert nurses derived from their experience and the way in which they developed intuition (Benner, 1984) and her work has had widespread impact on the way in which nursing knowledge is understood. The ethical basis of nursing has been well debated in many texts and papers, and although the use of aesthetics has largely been confined to teaching methods, it is probable that it may, in time, form an important part of nursing debates.

These developments can be attributed to an increasing awareness of the limits of traditional science. These limits are not simply consequences of particular methods and approaches, for example, the use of quantitative methods to study topics which are arguably better studied by using qualitative approaches. Whatever the approach chosen, research can only ask, answer or explore questions in a particular way. Research deals with observable and recordable events and occurrences, whether these be feelings or behaviours. It can seek to count the frequency of these events, describe them in detail, or seek to find links between events, and researchers pursue these aims in ways that are acceptable to their peers.

Nurses, however, have other types of questions to ask, which are not amenable to traditional research methods, and these are essentially philosophical questions. Moral philosophy, or ethics, of course has long been a concern of all health-care workers, and so there has been a tradition of conducting debates which lie outside research, but these debates are widening and involving other areas of philosophy.

The growth of philosophical ideas in nursing

An examination of current nursing journals is an indication that nurses are drawing on philosophy in their writing and thinking. Looking through the references given at the end of papers, it is not all that uncommon to find the names of philosophers such as Wittgenstein, Descartes and Heidegger being included. Sometimes these works are used to illuminate particular philosophical points about research methodology, and in this way provide a way of putting research into a philosophical context, but there is also an increasing number of papers which could be called 'philosophical discourses'. In other words, they do not involve the presentation of the result of empirical research, but are papers based on the presentation and discussion of arguments, which the author has linked to wider debates in philosophy.

One such example is the paper by Cash (1990) called 'Nursing models and the idea of nursing'. In this, the author challenges the notion that there is an 'essence' of nursing which, when detected, can distinguish nursing from non-nursing activity. This idea has, of course, been the basis of many attempts to define nursing or to construct nursing theories, most of which have had limited success. Cash compares this idea of things having an essence with the ideas of Wittgenstein, who was the catalyst for much of the philosophical work on language in this century. Wittgenstein suggested that although we may give things a name or a category, this does not necessarily mean that the name is a straightforward response to identification of a common element in them. The word 'game', for instance, is used to describe a number of activities which do not have a single common factor. Not all games involve competition, not all are fun, not all are physical, not all are unpaid, yet we still call them 'games'. The similarity between them, Wittgenstein suggests, is like a 'family resemblance'. People can be recognized as being part of the same family even though they do not all share a common feature or essence.

Wittgenstein suggests that many of our everyday classifications are based on such types of resemblance, and Cash suggests that this is the case with nursing. In other words, Cash's argument is that there is no essence of nursing, no single thing that all nurses do, but that nurses are recognizable through their 'family resemblance'. A nurse manager, a nurse in a cardiology unit, a nurse who is a health promoter and a nurse in a long-stay care of the elderly unit do not necessarily have any one activity in common, yet they are all recognizable as nurses.

Cash's paper is a good example of philosophy being used to explore nursing in a way that research cannot. It depends upon the careful analysis of contrasting ideas and arguments which are evaluated in terms of the logical justifications made for them. At the end of the paper, we have gained insight into a possible way of thinking about nursing which could change the way in which we would see the development of nursing theory. This type of critical examination of cherished assumptions is as valid and important as research which perpetuates or takes them for granted.

The areas in nursing that are ripe for philosophical enquiry are legion. To take a recent example of a debate in nursing and health care, there are the questions that are being raised about the nature of health-care provision. The model of health care that has become most dominant in the past decade in the UK, although it has been longer established in countries like the USA, is one based on market economics. Health care is therefore seen as a commodity to be purchased, and like other commodities, to be sold. This has directed political debate to consideration of marketing, consumer satisfaction, cost-effectiveness, and competitiveness – ideas which have been more common in the parlance of industry and commerce. This model is in direct conflict with other notions about health care, say, for example, that it is a right of all citizens, that it is a humane response of society to suffering, or even that it is a means by which a society can safeguard its future in the face of war or technological advances.

It is clear that these questions cannot be decided by research studies. It is impossible to imagine the research design which would allow researchers to conclude that health care is one or the other of these things. Research may be able to look at the impact of different models in terms of outcomes for patients and services, but it cannot, except in passing, tackle a question which might be more accurately understood as being about the metaphysics of health care.

Philosophy, however, has much to offer in this debate. Philosophical enquiry can take many forms, and focus on different aspects of the problem to hand, but if the question about the nature of health care were to be tackled, it would necessarily involve a closer inspection of the terms and concepts invoked in the debate. Notions such as 'consumer' and 'commodity' would be contrasted with 'patient' and 'service', and questions would be raised about the way in which these terms are being used and defined. Linked to this examination would be an inspection of the arguments used to justify the different positions taken in the debate. The idea that health care is a commodity to be bought and sold, like apples in a shop, would be scrutinized. Is an apple the same as a replacement hip? Is the agreement between shopkeeper and customer the same as that between doctor and patient? On what grounds are these claims to similarity being made, and how logical are these claims? How far do the similarities extend, and where do differences become apparent?

Having identified, disentangled and evaluated the various ideas that make up the argument, a philosophical enquiry could then look at how these ideas have been developed in other fields outside health care. The debate about the nature of health care may draw upon writing and thought in the areas of political philosophy, debates on justice, the nature of man, rights and duties, ethics and many other areas of philosophy, which both extend and clarify the debate. Ideas developed in other fields and at other times can be brought to bear upon current debates and their contribution evaluated.

What would the results of such an enquiry look like? Critics of philosophy would argue that at the end of this process we would be simply left with better defined concepts, and otherwise little further forward – there would be no 'facts' to go on. This type of criticism fundamentally misunderstands the purpose and nature of philosophy, which, indeed, to those eager for unequivocal declarations can seem like endless wordplay and navel-gazing.

If we were left 'only' with better defined concepts at the end of an examination of the marketing model of health care, many philosophers would argue that we had gained a great deal. Our ideas would be more rigorously developed, and we would not be tempted to casually pepper our arguments with jargon which was ambiguous in meaning. Through an examination of the words used in an argument, we can get a better idea of what is being advocated, and the logical implications of the positions being displayed. This seems to be a worthwhile achievement.

Philosophy can do more than clarify concepts, however. By examining the thinking which underpins concepts, and the arguments in which they are used, philosophical enquiry can begin to differentiate between sound and weak arguments, and identify those arguments which have firm logical foundations rather than those which do not. It might be possible, for example, that an examination of the humanistic model of health care would conclude that it is justified by arguments which do little more than appeal to mystical or sentimental notions of society, and that the difference made between apples and replacement hips is based on emotional appeals to the reader's sense of pity. Conversely, it could be argued that the fact that it is possible to appeal to pity indicates that this emotion is an important factor in the way that people prioritize things, and is therefore justified. That people can feel pity for someone who needs a replacement hip, but not so much for someone who 'needs' an apple (unless, of course, they are starving) suggests that there is a difference between the two needs.

It is, therefore, possible that two writers might reach different conclusions about the same question – a possibility which can infuriate many readers. Reading two such conflicting papers, it is difficult to escape the feeling that philosophy cannot tell us anything, and that it is all a matter of personal opinion. We are therefore justified in sticking to our own opinions because there is no way of telling which is right and which is wrong.

Dealing with conflicting opinions, however, is not a problem confined to philosophy. The same problem occurs in research, where two studies can have conflicting results. When faced with contradictory research findings, we immediately start to look at how they have been arrived at. We look at the research question, the sampling strategy, the methods used, and the analysis of data and we would usually conclude either that one study was stronger than another, and therefore to be more useful as an aid to under-standing, or we would conclude that the two studies could be synthesized to form a general statement with some qualifications, or that the two studies were different enough to stand alongside each other.

This is much the same way as conflicting philosophical arguments can be dealt with. Again, it would be possible to look at the questions asked and the methods used, and to regard them as either complementary or to decide that one paper makes a stronger case than the other. In carrying out this sort of analysis, therefore, we are engaged in philosophy ourselves, and our critical abilities are as much in evidence as they are when reading research. Philo-sophy cannot give us easy answers to our problems any more than research can, but if we understand its aims and methods, then we can use it creatively and critically to inform our thinking and action.

This discussion has tended to talk about 'Philosophy' as if it were some sort of tool which can be pulled off the shelf and used to sort out nursing. It is probably more accurate to think of philosophy as a range of tools that can help examine different problems, and so, like anyone who uses tools, it is important to understand the nature and capabilities of each one. In the next chapter, we will look at different philosophical methods which each have a particular tradition and have been used to examine different problems. It will be useful, therefore in this chapter, to give some background to these methods, and to describe the traditions that they come from.

A brief history of philosophy

An attempt to give a concise history of philosophical thought is bound to be superficial, and so we have included a list of further reading for those who wish to find out more. What we can do here, however, is to give a broad picture of some of the ideas that have been expounded and critiqued throughout history, and, most importantly, link them to events and thought in other areas. This is an important point to grasp, that philosophy does not go on as an activity separate from other happenings: that it is inextricably linked to the social context and the particular problems of the age. Social contexts give philosophy problems to consider and, particularly in the case of developments in science, new lines of thought to follow. In this way, developments in philosophy reflect and shape other areas of thought.

Before we begin this brief history of philosophy, another point should be noted, and that is that we will concentrate on Western philosophy, in other words the work of philosophers from Europe and North America. This is, in some ways, a narrow version of philosophy, which fails to address thoroughly the issues raised by philosophical traditions in the rest of the world, for example the Oriental philosophers, and the many writings available in Hindu and Buddhist traditions. This in part reflects our origins; as Westerners we are more familiar with Western philosophy, which has been the dominant form of philosophy available to us. It therefore makes some sense, in what is essentially an introductory text, to concentrate on the forms of philosophy which readers will be most likely to come across. We would not, however, suggest that Western philosophy is the only philosophy worth looking at, and we have listed some texts which might help readers who wish to explore philosophy further.

We have adopted a crude system of organizing this history, dividing philosophy into ancient, medieval, modern and contemporary periods. This has the virtue of being easy to grasp, but there is a danger that this structure might be interpreted to mean that there were abrupt changes marking the end of these periods, in the way that palaeontologists might mark the end of one Prehistoric period and the beginning of another. Even this cannot be done with precision, and in philosophy which deals with ideas which do not have clearly defined chronological periods of existence, it is even more difficult. Nor should a chronological structure be interpreted to mean that ideas or schools of thought existed and were then replaced by subsequent ideas. Such a quasi-evolutionary model of philosophy would suggest that say, in contemporary philosophy no-one discusses or even mentions the ancients, as their ideas are now redundant. We find, however, that the work of earlier philosophers is still the subject of much debate today – it has not become obsolete or redundant in the way that, say early theories of infection are in modern health care.

Ancient philosophy

What we know of ancient philosophers and their work is dependent upon the records and writings that have survived since their time, as much as the importance of their ideas. Discussions of ancient philosophy, therefore, tend to concentrate on the work of the Greeks and Romans, given that these philosophers have left records for us to examine. Literacy and education flourished in this era, and so it is not surprising that this is the case – another example of how philosophy relates to social contexts.

The social context of ancient philosophy is an interesting one. Science, as we know it today, was in its infancy, and so many of the attempts to understand the natural world proceeded by debate and argument, rather than empirical research. At the same time, the mystical descriptions of the nature of the world, derived from the myths and legends of the Gods, were losing influence, and the concern of the philosophers was to replace them with more rational and potentially verifiable explanations. This search for rational order was perhaps also influenced by the political climate of the time, where, while states enjoyed relatively lengthy periods of stability, they also faced problems of organization in peace time in order to preserve and protect their success and ensure the continuance of their society. The move of people from rural areas to cities also posed new problems of social order.

It is against this background that philosophers such as Socrates, Plato and Aristotle began to produce lectures and writing. They were not the first, or the only ancient philosophers, but their work has endured better than many others. Socrates is often credited with bringing the term 'philosophy' roughly translated as 'love of wisdom' into general parlance, as he constantly stressed that he did not possess wisdom, but was constantly striving for it. As a teacher, therefore, his approach was to challenge his listeners, and subject them to exhaustive questioning, rather than impart information, and it is his method of debate which has had such an impact on philosophy since. Much of our knowledge of Socrates is derived from the accounts of his lectures that Plato, one of his pupils, wrote, and probably added to, and so it is difficult to determine which are Socrates' ideas and which are Plato's.

In the work of Socrates and Plato, we find a concern with certainty and order, a possible reflection of the political disputes of the time, and an idea of knowledge as something that is recollected rather than discovered, which is understandable at a time when the natural sciences and their tools of discovery were in their infancy. These two themes have endured in various forms ever since in Western philosophy: a search for absolutes to be conducted through debate and questioning.

Plato, in his discussions on the nature of the world, and what we could know about it, developed the notion of forms or ideas, which were the essence of phenomena. For example, he argued that there was a pure form of beauty, and that all the things that we call beautiful, would evince this essence to some degree. The pure form, however, could never be apprehended directly – it could only be deduced by logical examination of the world. Plato's forms have left a legacy in philosophy and everyday thought which is difficult to shake off – we think of many things, such as truth, goodness or evil in this way. Another legacy is the accompanying dualism – that our senses provide limited and inaccurate information, and the only source of certainty is the mind and reasoning. This dualism manifests itself in the mistrust of the senses, and therefore the body that experiences sensations. As this is counterintuitive to the way that we live our lives – most of us are acutely aware of our bodies and of the things that we perceive around us, and base our decisions on them – the emphasis on the inner life can often seem irrelevant or appropriate.

Plato's ideas were, of course, challenged throughout the Ancient world, perhaps most notably by Aristotle, one of his pupils. Aristotle was much concerned with the physical world, and the world of nature, and it is to him that we owe the classification system of living things that we still use today. Aristotle argued against Plato's philosophy on the grounds that he presented forms as separate from the substance or matter that evinced them, a position that Aristotle found nonsensical. Whereas Plato argued that we could know of forms without directly experiencing them, Aristotle argued that knowledge comes from experience. For example Aristotle made a distinction between Universals and Particulars and argued that if there was a Universal of, say, red, it could not exist, and we could not know it apart from particular red things. Bertrand Russell described Aristotle as 'Plato diluted by common sense' further pointing out that this is a difficult combination as 'Plato and common sense do not mix easily'. In some ways this is true – if we take common sense to be the way in which ordinary people understand the world, then the writings of Plato seem to be of a quite different order. Aristotle's mixture of everyday experience and philosophical analysis is therefore sometimes very difficult to follow.

Aristotle's concern with the analysis of experience did not involve the rejection of logic; indeed, Aristotle spent much time in developing logic. In particular, he produced a logical form known as the syllogism, which was concerned with the logical relationship between classes of things and their characteristics. A famous form of the syllogism goes as follows:

All men are mortal   (Major premise)
Socrates is a man   (Minor premise)
Therefore Socrates is mortal   (Conclusion)

The syllogism, in its various formulations, has played an important part in logical debate since the time of Aristotle, and in the next chapter we will explore it further. What is important to note here is that there are many kinds of debate where the syllogism is not particularly useful, where the questions being asked are about the components of the syllogism itself rather than the relationship between them. Concentration on the syllogism as the primary form of logical argument severely restricts the kind of questions that can be debated, and so while it was useful for the sorts of debates that the Ancients were concerned with, it is not adequate in other ventures.

Medieval philosophy

Medieval philosophy is also related to the concerns and issues which faced society at the time, in particular the rise of Christianity. At the time most centres of learning were devoted to theology and the study of the Scriptures, which posed some problems of inconsistency. Medieval philosophy, therefore, was concerned with explaining and resolving the internal contradictions found in the Bible, and also with resolving the contradictions posed by the notion of an omnipotent, just, and good God, and the everyday experience of a life which was often brutal, violent and seemingly unjust.

An obvious way out of this dilemma was to argue that the material world was only a temporary state, and that all would be well in the afterlife. This turns human life into an opportunity for collecting merit awards through suffering, but it fails to answer doubts about a God who could create such a world – can a pure and good deity create evil, even as a sort of spiritual obstacle course?

These debates about the nature, capabilities and intentions of God occupied medieval philosophy for centuries. Philosophy was also affected by the work of the ancient philosophers as well, with philosophers drawing on the works of Plato in particular, as well as the Bible. Two of the most significant participants in this venture were St Augustine (AD 354–430) and St Thomas Aquinas (1225–74), representing early and late Christian medieval philosophy, and these two will serve as examples of some of the ideas that were developed during this period.

St Augustine tackled, amongst many other things, the nature of time. This arose from a concern with the question of what existed before God created the world, and indeed, what existed before God. Augustine's answer was that time began at the moment of creation, an answer that might be theologically tidy, but which raises many philosophical questions about the nature of time. What does it mean to say that 'time began' at such and such a point, and what sort of things could exist before it began? Augustine was therefore drawn on to an analysis of time which began with the way that we experience it, and the relationship between God and time. If God is eternal, Augustine argued, then God must exist in an eternal present – it makes little sense to talk about early or late eternity, because eternity is, by definition, impossible to apply chronology to.

Placing God outside of time leads Augustine to a relativistic view of time – contrasting the present with the past and the future. The past and the future happen, but only the present really *is*. Augustine therefore talks about the past as memory, and the future as expectation – both present phenomena. Memory and expectation are, however, subjective and essentially in the mind – ergo, time is a mental phenomenon. Augustine remained, however, humble in the knowledge that God knew everything, and did not presume to claim that he had solved the problem of time, instead portraying his work as incomplete and rudimentary. He therefore prayed to God to enlighten him further.

The omnipotence of God made some things unknowable in medieval philosophy, but it also provided a way out of tangled debates when philosophy ground to a halt. An argument could proceed up to a certain point, and when difficulties were encountered, the buck could be passed to God. This was not simply a cunning ploy to outwit opponents, or stifle debate, but a reflection of the power that the Church and Christianity had on philosophers and all other people. Scholarship, being largely theological, was for the glory of God, and most writers were inspired by a desire to worship and obey, rather than radically challenge the dominant and pervasive religious ethos that existed at the time. Philosophers therefore trod on dangerous ground if they claimed to have solved problems through their own thought rather than through Divine guidance, or if it was thought that they were doing so.

Things had not changed all that much by the end of the medieval period, in terms of the way that scholarship and philosophy were organized. There were, however, some changes in the Classical influences on philosophy, namely a move towards the writing of Aristotle and away from the work of Plato. St Thomas Aquinas, for example, persuaded the Catholic Church that Aristotle's philosophy would form a sounder basis for Christian theology than the works of Plato. While St Augustine had been a Platonist in as much as he had agreed with Plato's assertion that truth is not to be found by the perceptions of the senses, St Thomas Aquinas followed Aristotle's theory of causes as evidence of the existence of God. Aristotle had argued that things had several causes – the material cause, that things are the way they are because of the matter that they are made of, the formal cause, that things are the way that they are because of their form, the efficient cause, that things are the way that they are because of the way that they function, and the final cause, that things are the way that they are because of the end or aim that they have. For Aristotle and Aquinas, the final cause of all things is God.

Much of St Thomas's writing refers to the question of causality, in particular the cause of the world. Arguing that every event has a cause, and that this can be traced back to a prior cause indefinitely, Aquinas argued that there must be a first cause, and that this is God. The influence of Aristotle is also evident in other work of Aquinas' particularly when he uses sensory knowledge of the world in his arguments for the existence and nature of God. For example, he argues that the way that we can call both the sun and the heat generated by it 'hot', depends on the use of analogy. Analogy can also be used to understand God – using analogy of proportionality and analogy of attribution. Using the former, we can extend our knowledge of human wisdom, and apply these to God. It must be noted, however, that this does not work for baser human characteristics – we cannot attribute greed, for example, to God, because God is wholly good.

Modern philosophy: the Renaissance and the rise of science

The deliberations of the Christian philosophers were mainly concerned with explaining and understanding God, and although they may have strayed into science or nature, the touchstone was always God. As the Renaissance dawned, however, the stranglehold of religion weakened somewhat, and science and scientific methods were becoming more sophisticated, less speculative and more empirical. This did not mean, however, that philosophers abandoned speculation and logical analysis in favour of telescopes – the traditions of debate were firmly ingrained by now, and there was still the legacy of Platonic dualism which placed sensory knowledge in the realm of uncertainty. In the intellectual world of the time, therefore, there was a separation between those who studied the natural world (an area referred to for some time as 'natural philosophy') and those who continued the tradition of metaphysical debate. The division was by no means complete – many philosophers attempted to address the empirical world, and many scientists expressed their findings in metaphysical terms.

The work of the scientists was, however, having such an impact on the intellectual world that many long-cherished conclusions about the nature of life were being challenged, and in particular Christian beliefs. This gave philosophers new problems, which some of them saw as being about how to defend God against science. Some of them attempted to find a quasi-scientific basis for God, and still others sought to find logical rather than theological arguments for human conduct.

During this period, then, there were some re-enactments of the mind–body debate with conflicting positions expressed by the rationalists (for example, Descartes) and the empiricists (for example, Hume). This debate is covered in more detail in Chapter 3 on the philosophy of knowledge, so it is enough to say here that the concerns were, partly, to map out what it was possible for man (and science) to know. While Descartes argued that the ultimate source of knowledge was the mind, as sensory impressions were always suspect, the empiricists attempted to find a way of incorporating sensory data (which after all, was the basis of science) into discussions of knowledge. This proved extremely difficult to do, but it produced some interesting results. Hume, for example, produced an analysis of human reasoning about the empirical world, which bears significant resemblance to the modern-day discipline of psychology, arguing in particular that our notions of causality are simply because we mentally associate events with each other – we cannot really know that X causes Y, we simply expect them to follow each other. There is nothing about our sensory experience which shows us what the causal link is.

In addition to these debates about knowledge, there was also a debate about ethics or moral conduct, and again it is convenient (although a little simplistic) to think of this as a debate between the deontological or duty-based position of philosophers such as Kant, and the teleological or ends-based position of philosophers such as Mill. The details of these positions are explored further in Chapter 6 on moral philosophy, but it is worthwhile to note here that Mill and other utilitarians were proposing a system of ethics which was not religious in nature, and therefore were making a distinct contribution to ethical debate at a time when the edicts of the Church were losing their hitherto unquestioned authority.

It is also worth noting that Kant, in addition to developing a system of ethics, is also credited with bringing together, to some extent, the rationalist and empiricist positions on knowledge. This he did by arguing that the fact that the world is experienced, talked about, and known about, suggests that this world must satisfy certain conditions in order for it to be experienced. Here Kant distinguished between 'the world in itself' and the world of 'appearances', the former being the world as it is (and about which we can do nothing) and the latter the world as we experience it. Prior to Kant, it had been argued that there were only two kinds of propositions that could be made about the world: firstly analytic a priori statements, which were true by definition and known independently of evidence from the senses (such as all fathers are male) and secondly synthetic a posteriori statements, which required empirical evidence to support them (such as water boils at 100°C). Kant argued that there was a third class of statement, synthetic a priori statements (such as all events have a cause), which are conditions of our experience of the world of appearances. The task of philosophy, therefore, became for Kant the working out of these synthetic a priori statements, rather than a struggle between the validity of analytical a priori statements and synthetic a posteriori statements. This gave philosophers a means of seriously considering the world of appearances or sensory impressions, in a way that had not been possible before.

Contemporary philosophy

This century has seen a number of extremely interesting philosophical developments, belying any view that philosophy has run out of steam. Again, as in past periods, philosophy has developed against a background of changing social circumstances. This century has seen two world wars, the rise of secularism, the advent of popular culture, and, some would rather optimistically argue, the collapse of class structures.

EXISTENTIALISM

One of the interesting trends which can be observed in contemporary philosophy is the focus on experience, which in part was enabled or stimulated by Kant. This trend is, perhaps, most famously found in the writings of the existentialists, who have had a major impact on philosophy and art this century. Most discussions of existentialist philosophy begin with an apology for treating such a diverse group as a 'movement', given that such a classification tends to obscure the wide differences between the philosophers concerned. Having said this, however, the classification is useful, in that it emphasizes the concern that these philosophers had with the world of experience – life as it is lived, rather than life as it is thought about.

The roots of existentialist thought have been traced back to several philosophers, who were, interestingly, quite different in their backgrounds and aims. Kierkegaard, for example, was a Christian philosopher who reacted against the Hegelian notion of an objective science of human life. Kierkegaard argued that this obscured Christian faith, and its importance in human affairs, and disregarded subjective human experience which gives rise to faith. It is in his examination of the subjective experience of life that many ideas are found which were developed later by other existentialists, albeit without the emphasis on Christian faith. Husserl, on the other hand, did ascribe to the project of developing a systematic 'map' of human nature, and in particular the way in which the mind responds to experiences – an important aspect of this being the way in which the mind is directed towards experiences and objects. This directedness means that 'I can not only see a table', for example, but 'I can have beliefs about it, preferences about it, plans for it, and memories of it'. Husserl's extensive analysis of these responses was phenomenological in that it dealt with responses to phenomena, but Husserl did not devote much time to an examination of these phenomena, which he held could be entirely illusory – the important thing was not what had happened, but what the mind thought had happened. Consciousness was therefore the key to understanding the human mind, and experience was 'bracketed' in that questions about it were not pursued or asked. The exact nature of experience was not regarded as an interesting question to persue.

Husserl's concentration on the mind has echoes of the split between mind and body espoused by Descartes, and subsequent existentialists became increasingly dissatisfied with this, arguing that it relegated the world outside the mind to a series of illusions. Calling the empirical world into question in this way, or simply ignoring it, did little to progress the understanding of how people managed to live in it, and treat it as non-illusory. Husserl's notion that human existence was based on a subject–object relationship between the mind and the empirical world was challenged by one of his followers, Heidegger, who questioned this idea of our relationship to things. Heidegger argued that in much of life people do not have subjective experiences of objects, but in fact live much of their time without awareness or consciousness of objects, but still manage to use them and live with them. In reading a book, for example, the reader is not often conscious of the structure of the binding, the mechanisms of the pages, or the seat that is being sat on (unless, of course, the book is very boring, the binding clumsy, or the seat uncomfortable). The reader still, however, manages to read the book, turn the pages, and adjust the sitting position when necessary. Heidegger argued that for much of the time, the world of objects is 'transparent' to us. This observation further led Heidegger to argue that living is not about being a subject in a world of objects, but that we are 'in the world' and of the world (Heidegger used the term *Dasein* which can be translated as 'being there'). This was a radical view of what it is to be a person, which went some way to overturning the Cartesian legacy of dualism, which had led philosophers to variously try to find ways of validating the empirical world, or to dismiss it and regard life as a mental phenomenon. Heidegger argued that dualism was a false dichotomy – we simply are of the world that we experience. Even when we stand back to contemplate the world, we do so as part of it, with a shared background.

Heidegger's other contribution was to emphasize the importance of time, when he argued that much of our activities are directed towards aims. We read a book in order to gain understanding or pleasure, we use a hammer in order to make things, we sit on a chair in order to rest; Heidegger's argument goes beyond such short-term explicit goals, and suggest that our whole life is characterized by progress and movement. In such a view, time becomes an important element of life.

The problem with Dasein, as Heidegger saw it, was that it can lead to lives directed by conformity. Because we are so unaware, consciously, of the world, we can live our lives automatically, without thinking about what we are doing, or why we are doing it. If we do stop to think about it, we can become overwhelmed by the 'ungroundedness' of what we do and the lack of meaning that our lives have. When faced with this realization, we can either flee back to conformity, or try to live our lives differently, in a more 'authentic' way which is not hidebound by convention.

The notion of authenticity was one that was taken up enthusiastically by other existentialists, famously by Sartre. The idea that life was essentially meaningless, and that people should throw off convention was one that seemed increasingly powerful in the social unrest of the Second World War. Sartre, however, extended the idea of the meaninglessness of life to the extent where he became almost a neo-Cartesian, starting off with individual consciousness which he saw as completely free of convention and the world, and where we can give any meaning we like to the decisions that we make. This was not the view of Merleau-Ponty, another existentialist, who filled some of the gaps left by Heidegger in his discussions of the nature of the body and perception, which Heidegger had neglected. Merleau-Ponty's discussions emphasized the way in which life is embodied and how this directs our existence – we are not completely free.

PRAGMATISM

Another development in philosophy in the late nineteenth and early twentieth century which deserves a mention is the American school of pragmatism, which has had a significant influence on ideas about knowledge and learning. We discuss it in more detail in the chapter on the philosophy of knowledge, but here it deserves a mention as a contrast to existentialism. The American pragmatists, were, as the name suggests, interested in the practical consequences of ideas (the term 'pragmatism' comes from the Greek term for 'deed' or 'action'), but this was not simply a crude dismissal of ideas themselves. Their questions, about meaning, truth and knowledge, were sophisticated and complex, and their work has endured, in various forms, in politics, education and psychology.

To take one example; C.S. Pierce developed a maxim of meaning, which goes roughly as follows: our conception of an object is entirely about the effects that we perceive an object of our conception to have. Pierce here was arguing that our idea of an object is about what that object does, in other words that meaning must always relate to something that *happens*. It is therefore possible to verify meanings or terms, with reference to actions – if two things do the same thing, then they have the same meaning.

LANGUAGE

The above example of a pragmatic maxim illustrates an interest which much of contemporary philosophy shares – the interest in meaning, terminology and language. Heidegger's philosophy is difficult to read because of his language – the joining together of words to convey new ideas is difficult to translate into English. However, his creative use of language reflects one of his chief concerns, i.e. the way in which language can help to reflect, promote and stabilize new ideas and ways of being. The pragmatists were also concerned with language in their debates on meaning, although they seemed to adopt a stance which looked at the 'accurate' matching of terms with ideas.

This view of language as a matching of words to things was also a concern of the logical positivists at the beginning of this century, who essentially treated language as a system of logic, and therefore amenable to logical analysis. One of the contributors to this movement was Wittgenstein, with the publication of his *Tractatus Logico-philosophicus* in which he argued that language has the purpose of stating facts, and because it can do so, it must have a logical structure. It is therefore possible to imagine a perfect language, unambiguous, clear and logical, with which we can state facts. Other areas of life, which are not facts, are not amenable to this type of analysis, and therefore Wittgenstein concludes that 'Whereof we cannot speak, thereof we must be silent'.

Wittgenstein, however, developed his ideas in quite a different direction, following the *Tractatus*, and came to concentrate on language use rather than language structure. He talked about language as a game, with rules, and as something which, although it did not map onto the world in a direct way, was still understood by all. Language does a variety of things, not just stating facts, but because we still partly believe in the notion of language as fact-stating, we tend to become confused about other games. In the game of wishing, for example, we may think of the wishes uttered as mapping onto some sort of psychological fact about ourselves – a fundamental mis-understanding of the game. Realizing what we do with language, and how we do it, Wittgenstein argues, puts many 'philosophical problems' in their place.

POST-MODERNISM

This interest in language, and the way in which it is used is at the heart of post-modernism. This development in philosophy (although it is also a development in architecture, art and literature) has been expounded largely by philosophers such as Derrida and Lyotard, and partly due to its recent notoriety, has become almost a compulsory element in any contemporary conversation that aspires to be intellectual. 'Post-modernism' was a term first used in architecture to describe a rejection of modernism (not surprisingly!) in which buildings were designed according to technological and functional criteria. In philosophy, the term came to mean a cynicism about and deconstruction of 'meta-narratives' about society, for example Marxism. Such modernist portrayals of history suggested a progress of human society through scientific and rational analysis and development. The analysis will reveal the 'deep structure' of the world. In fact post-modern thinkers recommend that the whole search for deep, universal truths, which underlie ordinary life, and which seems to them to have characterized intellectual enquiry since the Enlightenment has to be abandoned. There are no universal truths, no foundations which shore up, say our aesthetic preferences, our scientific investigations or our moral judgements.

The post-modernist project is to show that analysis does not reveal any monolithic truth about the world, but heterogeneity, culturally constructed difference and impermanence. Foucault's analysis of medicine is an example of a post-modern approach, which challenges the modernist notion of the progression of medicine through the acquisition of skills and knowledge. Foucault argues that medicine has progressively 'colonized' areas of human life which were originally thought of as outside the remit of medicine, and what we take now to be 'medical' is socially constructed.

This general style of thinking reaches its limit in the work of Derrida. Derrida's deconstruction of texts attempts to show how certain terms come to be 'privileged' and others 'marginalized'. Derrida argues, however, that such a process is ultimately mistaken – for every set of binary terms, such as internal/external or good/evil, the privileged term can only make sense in conjunction with its opposite – it is parasitic on it. Paying attention to the way in which terms and ideas are marginalized or privileged reveals no deep structure, simply a series of choices. One obvious objection to this way of thinking is that these too are claims, true or false, about the nature of our relation to language and to the world. Why is post-modernism exempt from the recommended abandonment of the 'search for truth'? The post-modern answer to this objection is the development of a peculiar and to many irritating style of writing in which claims are advanced just sufficiently to be withdrawn by an endless series of qualifications, undercuttings and change of direction. For this reason, among others, the newcomer to philosophy does better to understand the tradition to which post-modernism is a reaction rather than to dive straight into the works of post-modern writers.

FEMINISM

The observant reader may have noticed that all the people mentioned in this brief history are men. This is perhaps due to the fact that it is only comparatively recently that women have been a part of the academic world, and therefore have not been able to enter into the formal debates and writing that make up an orthodox history of philosophy. Now that women are entering the world of formal philosophy, however, they are highlighting and critiquing the limitations of the male perspective.

The criticisms that feminist philosophers level against traditional philosophy are about the nature of the topics that it has been concerned with, the way that they are defined, and the way that it has tried to pursue them. Firstly, there is a critique of the over-cerebral delineation of problems, which has focused on problems of logic, rather than living. Feminist philosophers have argued that this focus has tended to dismiss the body in favour of the mind, and alongside this there has been a distaste for the physical. Moreover, the physical has been associated with women from the time of the Ancient Greeks, who regarded women as intellectually incapable of entering into any proper debate, trapped as they were by their animal, physical natures. Feminists would therefore argue that there is implied in the concentration on the intellect, a dismissal of women.

Philosophical method has also been critiqued by feminists, who have argued that the language of debate is adversarial. Setting up opposing positions and 'defending' them certainly seems to imply that only one position might prevail, whereas philosophy might be better served by a synthesis of the two. Attempts to develop a different form of philosophical discourse, however, run into many problems, partly because challenging traditions of debate is in itself an adversarial move, and a refusal to make the challenge is simply not recognized as philosophy. In addition, there is also the argument made by traditional philosophers, which is that if two arguments are contrasted with each other, the best way to decide between them is to have their weak points exposed – philosophy is not about philosophers being nice to each other, and to have a situation where philosophers simply politely defer to each other would result in a discipline without movement or change.

Despite these problems with method, feminist philosophers have been successful in changing the debates in philosophy to some extent, although whether this is entirely due to them, or whether things would have changed anyway is a moot point. Contemporary philosophical writing now tends to incorporate everyday experiences into debates, and references to such experiences often form the starting point for debate.

Philosophy and nursing – the possibilities

It can be seen from this brief account of philosophy, that it has always been tied to the social world in which it has taken place. This seems a very commonplace observation, but when Bertrand Russell first published his

History of Western Philosophy, critics made much of the fact that he had linked the history of philosophy with the social history of the cultures in which philosophers lived. Presumably until then philosophy had been viewed as having no temporal, geographical or social dimensions.

What has not been made clear in this account has been the impact of philosophy on other areas of life. To detail this would take the rest of the book, so it is perhaps enough to discuss here the impact of philosophy on nursing. Sometimes this impact is not at first obvious, nor is it always easy to trace ideas back to their origin, but there are some developments in nursing which have clear links to philosophical ideas. Most of these are with modern philosophy, especially the existentialist movement, which has given new directions to nursing research in particular. Phenomenology, a research approach which has gained in popularity over the past decade, was a fundamental part of the existentialist project which was to understand life as it is experienced, in an immediate and direct way. Nursing is very much an experiential occupation, in which the day-to-day phenomena of practice have great import and significance. The phenomena of nursing are not just those experienced by the nurse, but also by patients and clients, and their experiences of pain, suffering, joy and relief, are striking. It is not surprising, therefore, that phenomenology and the existentialist view of the human condition have been employed in understanding nursing.

Nurses also, however, work by principles as well as responding to phenomena, and so there is a great deal of nursing literature on values and ethics. Some of these debates can be traced back to the work of deontologists, such as Kant, and utilitarians, such as Mill, and conflicting ethical views often reflect the conflict between observing the right action and aiming for the right consequences. At another level, however, nursing ethics is also influenced by the existentialist notion of 'authenticity', being true to oneself, and helping others to do likewise. The fact that philosophy has not sorted out, once and for all, the ethical problems of nursing, is a good illustration of the way in which philosophy can be used. In ethical dilemmas, it can sharpen up the issues, lead to closer examination of situations, and link these to a wider debate. That it cannot tell us what to do, however, has been seen by some as philosophy's redundancy – unlike science, philosophy can only raise rather than answer questions.

In education, nursing has been influenced by many of the philosophical debates about the nature of knowledge. Again, there is the existentialist phenomenological approach evident in many teaching techniques which use critical incidents as a means of learning about nursing, and where the phenomena of practice are brought into the classroom. This approach is interesting in the way that it seeks to bridge the theory–practice gap, a concern of nursing which could be traced back to the mind–body division found in dualism. In education, we also find some influences from the American pragmatists, with their concentration on knowledge as being 'what works'.

In nursing practice, we find many ideas which can be linked back to philosophical ideas. In the way that nurses manage and organize their work we find many concepts, about justice, needs and rights, which have formed the debates in political philosophy. In direct care, we find ideas about holism, human potential and what it is to be human, which again can be traced back to philosophy. An interesting point here is whether some of nursing's ideas come from 'real' philosophers or not. Rogers, for example, was ostensibly a psychologist, but many of his ideas about human potential rest on well-argued logical grounds rather than empirical evidence, and as such seem more like philosophy. In our dealings with others, particularly as a predominately female profession, feminist issues come to the fore. Again, much of the writing is not necessarily presented as philosophy, but its nature is such that it seems very like it. Perhaps this indicates that philosophy happens in many places, and is not the sole province of 'qualified philosophers' (whatever they may be).

The question that must be asked is whether there is a philosophy of nursing. This is much the same debate which has occurred in science, where nursing uses theories from biology, chemistry, sociology and psychology. This issue of whether there will ever be a unified science of nursing, rather than the wholesale borrowing from other sciences, is similar to the debate about a nursing philosophy. Will nursing continue to borrow bits of ethics, and bits of logic, and bits of every other school, or will a new and unique branch of philosophy develop?

The answer depends on how a branch of philosophy is defined. If it is defined in terms of its subject matter, then it is perfectly possible for a philosophy of nursing to develop. If it is defined in terms of its metaphysical concerns, then this is less clear – it is difficult to think of the metaphysics of nursing as being very different from everybody else's, particularly as nursing is concerned with everybody else. If a philosophy of nursing emerges as a distinct branch of philosophy, however, this does not mean that it will not incorporate relevant and useful work done elsewhere. To reject this work would be the equivalent of rejecting knowledge about the circulation of the blood in nursing science – it would produce a body of thought which was not suited to its purpose. For this reason, we would argue that the best foundation for any potential philosophy of nursing is a clear understanding of other philosophy.

References

Benner, P. 1984: *From novice to expert*. Menlo Park, CA: Addison-Wesley.
Carper, B. 1978: Fundamental patterns of knowing in nursing. *Advances in Nursing Science*, **1**(1), 13–23.
Cash, K. 1990: Nursing models and the idea of nursing. *International Journal of Nursing Studies* **27**(3), 249–58.
Henderson, V. 1982: The nursing process – is the title right? *Journal of Advanced Nursing* **7**, 103–9.
Report of the Committee on Nursing. 1972: Cmnd 5115 (the Briggs Report). London: HMSO.

Further reading

Ayer, A.J. 1982: *Philosophy in the twentieth century.* London: Weidenfeld and Nicolson.

Benhabib, S. and Cornell, D. (eds) 1987: *Feminism as critique.* Oxford: Polity.

Emmet, E.R. 1965: *Learning to philosophise.* Harmondsworth: Pelican.

Fox, N.J. 1993: *Postmodernism, sociology and health.* Buckingham: Open University Press.

Frazer, E., Hornsby, J. and Lovibond, S. 1992: *Ethics: a feminist reader.* Oxford: Blackwell.

Gould, C. (ed.) 1983: *Beyond domination: new perspectives on women and philosophy.* Totowa, NJ: Rowman and Littlefield.

Janssen-Jurreit, M.L. 1982: *Sexism: the male monopoly on history and thought.* London: Pluto Press.

Jencks, C. 1992: *The post-modern reader.* Academy Editions.

Magee, B. 1982: *Men of ideas – some creators of contemporary philosophy; dialogues with fifteen leading philosophers.* Oxford: Oxford University Press.

Nagel, T. 1989: What does it all mean? – a very short introduction to philosophy. Oxford: Oxford University Press.

Russell, B. 1985: *History of western philosophy.* London: Unwin.

Sherwin, S. 1993: *No longer patient: feminist ethics and medicine.* Temple University Press.

Urmson, J.O. and Ree, J. 1989: *The concise encyclopaedia of western philosophy and philosophers.* London: Unwin Hyman.

Vesey, G. 1974: *Philosophy in the open.* Milton Keynes: Open University Press.

2 Logic, argument and reason

Introduction

This chapter is about the methodology of philosophy, i.e. the way in which philosophy investigates problems and reaches conclusions. Some of you may wish to skip this chapter, and if you decide to do so, it should not seriously affect your reading of the rest of the book. We would, however, suggest that you do spend some time on it, because it does give some context to the arguments presented elsewhere, and where the components of these arguments are not necessarily made explicit. Reading this chapter, therefore, should make it possible for you to examine the logic of other chapters in a more critical way. A critical stance is a very useful position to adopt, and one which sometimes appears lacking in nursing debates, where the rhetoric of patient care can silence objectors. Nurses, perhaps because they feel beleaguered in a world which does not appreciate or recognize them, have tended to aim for solidarity and consensus rather than dispute and difference, an understandable move, but one which can be unproductive in developing new ideas or challenging old ones.

Argument is the currency of philosophy. This does not mean that when we ordinarily disagree and remonstrate with one another, we are really doing philosophy, though we are often expressing beliefs, supporting judgements and giving reasons which form the raw material for philosophy. Nor does it mean that philosophy is a matter of violent disagreements, though philosophers do often passionately care about their ideas and theories. What it does mean is that, while outside of philosophy we are interested in someone's ideas and opinions simply because they are that person's ideas and opinions, in philosophy there is little interest simply in someone's opinion for its own sake. Rather, philosophers are interested in how people try to *support* their beliefs and *justify* their positions and claims. In assessing arguments, the philosophical tradition has developed an elaborate vocabulary with which to describe kinds of arguments, the components of arguments and the relation between those components. The higher reaches of this discipline – logic – need not concern us, but in this chapter we explain some of the basic ideas and how these are relevant to the practical examination of arguments. We also try to give some advice on how to avoid the kind of arguments that everyone finds tiresome and exasperating.

First of all, what is an argument? What we do not mean by this term here is a row in which Smith disagrees with Jones, Jones calls Smith a fool and Smith goes off in a huff (though logicians have been known to behave this way!). In fact, the term 'argument' has at least two different senses, both of which are important:

- An argument can be a dispute between two or more people in which some members of the group try to convince the others to adopt another position, to change their minds or to take some action. What distinguishes this from just a fight is that the participants seek to offer reasons for their claims which they hope the others will accept or they make reasoned objections to the claims which others are making. In this sense, an argument is an essentially social event or process.

- An argument is also a set of statements purporting to establish some particular claim. The argument might be found in a book, or in the back of one's mind or be at large in the culture. We will first examine this second sense of argument and then return to examining arguments in a social context. So, what, in this second sense, is an argument?

Recognizing arguments

How can we recognize arguments?

The way to answer this question is to ask what arguments are made of. A standard answer is that an argument is composed of linguistic entities – which we can call 'statements' or else 'propositions'. Examples of simple propositions are 'The weather is poor today', 'Brian is hungry' and 'The postmen are on strike'. But it should be obvious that there can also be much more complicated propositions such as 'If it is raining, then either the cat will come home or he will shelter in the bin and if he shelters in the bin, he will come back dirty when the rain stops'.

Premises and conclusions

Is an argument just a list of propositions then? No. An argument is a set of propositions in which the propositions are made to play particular roles. Propositions can play the role of premises or the role of conclusions. For example, the following argument contains three propositions:

1. All tigers are ferocious
2. Khan is a tiger

Therefore   3. Khan is ferocious

Propositions 1 and 2 are premises. Proposition 3 is a conclusion, drawn from the premises.

When analysing arguments, be sure to distinguish between the premises and the conclusions of arguments. Note also:

- A premise in one argument may have formed the conclusion of a previous argument.

- A conclusion in one argument may form a premise in a subsequent argument.
- Premises are *stated*, conclusions are *drawn* or *argued for*.

Truth and validity

- Truth (or falsity) is a property of propositions, not of arguments, Propositions can be true or false: arguments *cannot* be true or false.
- Validity (or invalidity) is a property of arguments, not of propositions or points. An argument is valid if the conclusion follows from the premises. An argument is invalid if the conclusion does *not* follow from the premises.

The term 'valid' often causes confusion. Outside of philosophy, it is perfectly correct to say that Smith has a valid point of view or that so and so made a valid point. What this means, roughly, is that Smith's views are deserving of consideration and respect or that so and so made a quite interesting point. Within science, people often talk about valid or invalid measurements or methods or even instruments. This means something like that the measurement or method or instrument meets the accepted scientific standards. It is sometimes used in philosophy; however, the term is (mostly) reserved for this specialized sense – a particular relation between premises and conclusions in an argument.

- Consequently, truth (or falsity) and validity (or invalidity) are independent of one another. An argument can be entirely composed of true propositions and yet still be an invalid argument. Conversely, an argument can be entirely composed of false propositions and still be valid.
- An argument which has true premises *and* is valid is called a sound argument.
- An argument which either has one or more false premises *or* is invalid is an unsound argument.

For example:

	1. All ducks can swim
	2. Donald is a duck
Therefore	3. Donald can swim

In this case:

- The premises are true.
- The argument is valid – the conclusion follows from the premises.
- So, the argument is sound

Consider the argument:

	1. All ducks can swim
	2. Donald is a duck
Therefore	3. Donald can fly

In this case:

- The premises are true and the conclusion is true.
- The argument is invalid – the conclusion does not follow from the premises.
- So, the argument is unsound.

Now consider:

        1. All ducks can type
        2. Donald is a duck
Therefore   3. Donald can type

In this case:

- One premise (the first premise) is false. The other premise is true.
- The argument is valid – the conclusion follows from the premises. Note that the argument is valid, even though one of the premises is false.
- So, the argument is unsound.

Finally, consider:

        1. All ducks can play squash
        2. All squash players can type
Therefore   3. All ducks can type

In this case:

- Both premises are false.
- The argument is valid – the conclusion follows from the premises. Note that the argument is valid, even though both premises are false.
- So, the argument is unsound.

The distinction between truth and validity *is absolutely fundamental in philosophy*. Why is this? As we have seen, philosophy is not a kind of very general empirical science. Consequently, the empirical truth or falsity of statements is rarely of much direct importance in philosophical argument. This does not mean that philosophers can safely hide in their armchairs from unpalatable facts. It does mean that philosophy is mostly interested in questions for which there is not or could not be any empirical evidence one way or another. Translating this point into the language of argument means that the truth of premises, and certainly the truth of conclusions, is less important in philosophy than the relation between the premises and the conclusions. Philosophers are, or ought to be (or used to be), interested in what is true. But their method of getting there depends heavily on assessing, not the truth of premises, but the validity of arguments. Hence it is always more useful in philosophy to consider the validity of arguments rather than the truth of fact describing statements. Consequently, it is very important that in the analysis of arguments – in deciding whether an argument is sound or unsound – we distinguish between:

- Agreeing or disagreeing with the truth of premises and conclusions.
- Agreeing or disagreeing that the argument is valid.

Conditional statements

Some arguments are conditional, in other words they predict or postulate states of affairs if certain conditions are met. This makes them quite complex to evaluate, because not only do the propositions and conclusions need to be examined , but also the soundness of the predictive part of the argument. Here are two examples to show how conditional arguments can be presented:

- If he drank too much last night, he had a headache this morning and he did drink too much last night. So we can conclude that he has a headache this morning.

- If he drank too much last night, he had a headache this morning and he did have a headache this morning. So we can conclude that he drank too much last night.

The structure of these arguments can be formulated in this way:

If P then Q
or
If *antecedent* then *consequent*

As in the examples of argument given earlier, it is possible to break down the argument into parts, in this case antecedent and consequent, and either affirm or deny them. The results of doing this are contained in Fig. 1. These kinds of arguments are often woven together into quite complicated chains made more complicated by a wide vocabulary for expressing them. Words like 'unless', 'without', 'should', etc. need translating into 'if . . . then' if we have any doubt about the validity of the argument in which they occur. For

AFFIRM THE ANTECEDENT	P THEREFORE Q	VALID
DENY THE CONSEQUENT	NOT Q THEREFORE NOT P	VALID
AFFIRM THE CONSEQUENT	Q THEREFORE P	INVALID
DENY THE ANTECEDENT	NOT P THEREFORE NOT Q	INVALID

Figure 1 Breaking down the argument into the antecedent and consequent to affirm or deny.

example, if someone is arguing 'P unless Q', then this needs to be reformulated as 'if Q then not P'. Similarly, 'P only if Q' has to be translated as 'if not Q then not P'.

'If . . . then' arguments are frequently used, and commonly misused. Sometimes the conditional nature of the argument is not appreciated by either the person who makes the argument or the person who hears it. If you make a conditional argument without realizing it, or having thought it through carefully, then you can be easily demolished by objections to either the antecedent or to the consequent. Alternatively, not spotting a conditional argument leaves you justifying unnecessarily. Thinking about conditional arguments, however, is mind-sharpening in the way that it leads you to examine the components of statements.

Inductive arguments

We have said that if an argument which is valid and which has true premises can be regarded as sound. However, it does not follow from this that all sound arguments must be valid arguments. In fact, every day we use sound arguments that, strictly speaking, are invalid. Consider the following argument:

> People who have taken higher than average levels of aspirin have lower than average risk of heart disease.
> So:
> If I take higher than average levels of aspirin then I will have a lower than average risk of heart disease.

Formally, this argument is invalid. That is, the conclusion does not follow from the premise. Indeed, there even seems to be important premises missing. Still, to most of us, it looks like an argument that we can find persuasive, and can act upon, given the truth of the premise. In fact, most of the arguments that we use and are persuaded by, most of the patterns of reasoning we engage in, are strictly speaking invalid. But that does not mean that these are unsound arguments. Rather they are sound examples of another type of argument; they are sound, *inductive*, as opposed to deductive, arguments.

There are a number of ways to describe inductive arguments. We can say that inductive arguments move from claims about a sample to claims about something which is not a member of the sample. Or we can say that inductive arguments move from claims about what we have so far experienced to claims about what we have not yet experienced or could not experience. Characteristically, the inductive process is as follows:

1 All the facts are observed and recorded in a totally impartial manner.

2 The observed facts are analysed and classified.

3 From this analysis, generalizations are drawn about the relations between the facts.

We move from 'the phenomena we are interested in and have observed are thus and so' to 'all the phenomena we could observe are thus and so'. Note that seen in this light, deductive arguments appear remarkably uninformative. For all we are doing in the conclusions of these deductive arguments is bringing out the implications of the premises. But in inductive reasoning, by contrast, we seem to be moving towards new and substantial knowledge. This is why it is so often claimed that real science must involve both inductive and deductive reasoning; inductive reasoning to generate testable hypothesis and deductive reasoning to carry out the tests.

Of course, not all inductive arguments are sound arguments. Some are altogether unsound. Compare:

'Every day of my life until now I have woken up feeling irritable.'
So:
'I will wake up feeling irritable tomorrow morning.'

'Every day of my life until now I have been under forty years of age.'
So:
'I will always be under forty years of age.'

The first argument is perfectly acceptable. If someone really had woken up feeling irritable every day of his life, then it would certainly be reasonable for him to accept that this will happen again tomorrow. But the second argument is not at all reasonable. It is unsound. Why? Not because it is invalid. As we have said, all inductive arguments are invalid. So what is wrong with it? Well, it flies in the face of all our experience. We know it must be wrong. In fact, there is no quite general way, as there is in the case of deductive arguments, of saying what makes an inductive argument unsound. We cannot just look at the form of the argument and determine its soundness. We have to look at its content and the relation of this content to our experience at large. We all know that the waking up in particular moods is just a different kettle of fish from getting older. But no formal rules can tell us. Inductive reasoning allows us to develop new knowledge about the world but the price we pay for this is the lack of precise rules to distinguish sound inductive arguments from unsound ones.

Some popular fallacies

Outside of the philosopher's logic lab, detecting poor arguments is less a science of precise rules but is more akin to judgements of character. One can be right or wrong but there are few hard-and-fast rules. Some arguments, like some character types, tend to turn up more often and most often when least welcome. It is useful then to be able to recognize these types. Philosophers call these particularly recognizable types of unsound argument, *fallacies*. Because arguments do not occur in a vacuum but are used to do things, very often the point of these fallacious arguments is to influence belief in order to bring about or prevent change of some sort. Here, as generally, the existence of fallacies is a function of the social and political context of arguments. Here are some common types that it is well worth learning to spot. As a useful exercise you might try remembering or constructing your own examples of each fallacy to put alongside these.

Name	Description	Example
The progress fallacy	Developments and changes are inevitably good things.	'There were people who said privatizing telephones wouldn't work. It did. There were people who said privatizing electricity wouldn't work. It did. And now they say that privatizing health care won't work!'
The 'one-way' fallacy	Given one premise, there is only one possible conclusion to be drawn, and generally applied.	'Why should an OAP living in the house she worked for all her life pay the same money as the five professionals next door? It's obvious that local government revenue should be on a per capita basis.'
The rhinoceros fallacy	If others agree to something, it is foolish to be left behind.	'All the other European countries are in favour of a single currency. So Britain should put aside its reservations and get on the EMU train.'
The slippery-slope argument	Once one small move is made, further moves, to the extreme, are inevitable.	'If we allow voluntary euthanasia, we'll end up with involuntary euthanasia.'
The 'no problem' argument	If there are no complaints or objections apparent, then there is no problem.	'The number of complaints about waiting time in casualty wards went down this month. We can be sure that the changes have proved popular.'
The 'practical man' argument	Something can be quite alright in theory but just wrong in practice so there is no need to examine the cogency of the theory.	'Letting patients have a say in care is a silly idea – it doesn't work in practice.'
The 'worse evil' argument	We should be concerned with worse evils, to the exclusion of other problems.	'Resources spent on smokers would be better spent on those who become ill through no fault of their own.'

The 'tradition' argument	Things that are traditional should be maintained simply because they are traditional.	'I don't know what these young doctors are complaining about. As a young houseman, I used to work 110 hours a week. Now I'm a successful consultant so it didn't do me any harm.'
Argumentum ad baculum	Arguing that an argument is valid by reference to the strategies which could be used to impose it.	'Management will recognize the justice of our claim when they reflect that we maintain the right to take industrial action.'
Argumentum ad hominem	Referring to a person's role or personality, etc. to explain or assume their position in an argument.	'You're bound to support long hours for doctors. Administrators don't know they're born!'
No true Scotsman move	Arguing that exceptions to a rule we support or counterexamples to a claim that we make are, by definition, not genuine exceptions or counterexamples.	'This survey showing that 10% of consultants prefer dealing with cases involving lucrative minor surgery to cases which take a lot of their time is nonsense. But no true consultant would put money ahead of medical need.'
Argument from respect	Arguing that certain positions are true or false because of the general characteristics of selected people who hold them.	'Pacifism is not irrational. Einstein was a pacifist and he could hardly be called irrational.'
The genetic fallacy	A thing is really only what its function is or what brought it into being.	'Man is just a survival machine for the transmission of genetic material.'
The sorites (heap) fallacy	Small incremental differences never amount to a big difference. Since a single grain of sand does not make a heap and since adding one more does not make a heap out of what is not a heap, there are no heaps of sand.	'One cigarette won't make a difference.'

The fat oxen fallacy	He who drives fat oxen must himself be fat – in other words, that it is possible to assume characteristics by association.	'If you want your skin to look natural, then use Brand X, made without any artificial additives.'
Fallacy of composition	It is possible to transpose the characteristics of individual elements to the whole group. What is true of the parts is true of the whole made up by the parts.	'All individuals pursue their own interests and these frequently come into conflict. Since individuals make up societies, it not surprising that there are clashes of interest between different societies.'
Fallacy of division	It is possible to transpose the characteristics of the whole group to its individual elements. What is true of the whole is true of the parts making up the whole.	'Iraq has shown its contempt for international law. So no Iraqi citizen can be trusted.'
Post hoc ergo propter hoc	Arguing that because A occurred after B, A occurred because of B.	'Since the abolition of the death penalty in Britain, the number of murders has sharply increased. So refusing to sentence murderers to death means signing a death warrant for the innocent instead.'

Practical strategies in argument

We have seen that an argument is a set of statements with any number of premises and one conclusion. Premises are statements which entail or support a conclusion. A statement can be a conclusion in one argument and a premise in another. What does this mean in practice? How should one conduct arguments?

It goes without saying that arguments should not be thought of as personal disputes in which the moral character of the people involved as well as the character of the issues is under attack. This does not mean that one should not care, that one has to suspend personal judgement, commitment or care about the issues. Philosophical argument is not a kind of complicated game for the emotionless. It does mean that, as well as being personally engaged in the argument, one keeps one eye on the structure of what is going on and takes regular opportunities to analyse the progress of the argument. Remarks like 'OK, I don't believe that you can establish that claim but what if I accept it for now. What follows?' or 'I can see that I'm not going to convince you this way so let me try another tack' help to establish the structure of the discussion and to help it go forward. Some more ideas for conducting arguments:

1 When trying to establish a conclusion, find out if and why there is dissent. Disagreement in conclusion is usually dependent upon disagreement about premises. But in philosophical disputes, it is also a matter of what is taken to follow from those premises given that they are true.

2 Make hidden premises explicit. Explicating premises involves working out what would establish the conclusion with which you disagree and what would have to be true for you to be wrong.

3 Do not burden another with stronger conclusions or premises than they wish to establish. If someone wants to establish that some doctors are selfish, do not hear the conclusion as 'all doctors are selfish'.

4 Do not accept stronger premises than you need to take you through your argument or try to establish stronger conclusions than you need. It is easy to feel that the bigger the conclusion the better. Conclusions which look very general and comprehensive seem very impressive. But philosophy is already working at a quite general level. So, within philosophy it is usually better to avoid the grand conclusion in favour of the more modest and specific point.

5 Beware of shifting premises and shifting conclusions. In the middle of a discussion, it is easy to forget what is under dispute or what is already agreed.

6 Ask whether the premises have to be accepted. Do we have to start from here?

7 Remind yourself of the point of what you are doing.

8 Remember that taking others along with you involves understanding and addressing their assumptions as well as your own.

9 Typically, a poor discussion is one in which:

   • More and more general statements have to be defended in order to sustain one or more of the conclusions. What begins as a dispute about necessary limits on patient choice ends up as a dispute about the limits of democracy given that people voted for this government which pushed through these changes to the health-care system

   • More and more issues are brought into play and the discussion moves to and fro between them.

   • There is frequent recourse to appeals to supposed authorities which then themselves come under dispute.

10 To counter this spiral, use the following strategies:

- Make frequent reviewing remarks so that it becomes clear when the argument has lost its focus or focused elsewhere. Take time to restate the original problem.
- Make sure that you ask questions as well as put forward your own answers:

  'What makes you say that?'
  'What do you think follows from that?'
  'Is that the same point as the one you made before or a different one?'
  'How do you think that counters the point I've just made?'
  'What do you think we've established so far?'
  'Since we're not going to reach agreement about that point, what's the next most important point we disagree about?'

11 Try to treat arguments as common pursuits. This is not a pious counsel of perfection. An argument is less likely to be productive for all concerned if protagonists become entrenched in their positions and feel that their personal standing is at stake. Avoiding this means keeping at least part of one's mind on the overall direction of the discussion as well as paying particular attention to the point presently under discussion.

Conclusion

This chapter has outlined the basics of the classical model of logic and argument. It can seem like always obeying the rules of logic is an impossible ideal. We may feel that none of us could be completely rational. Even if it were achievable, we may think, there would be concomitant costs, so that none of us would want to be completely rational. We are simply not intelligent enough always to see the logical consequences of our beliefs so that we are never inconsistent. Only, we might think, some kind of machine could be like this. But if we were like this, then we might have to forego emotion in becoming like a machine. Popular culture is keen to preach the message that our fallibility is loveable. In the *Star Trek* series, Mr Spock and his fellow Vulcans are supposed to be completely logical beings, but the price that they pay for this is the eradication of emotion, humour and insight. If this is right, why bother with reason at all? This involves a misunderstanding of the place of reason. Mr Spock's life is not just cold, arid and efficient – it is unintelligible. Logic gives us the rules for moving validly from statement to statement, premise to conclusion. What it cannot do is give us statements to believe, premises to start from. In order to have something to reason about, Mr Spock needs to have desires, interests, needs. Not even experience on its own could supply him with anything to which to apply his formidable logical powers. Why should he find an experience more or less interesting than another, unless he already has interests, desires or needs?

What this means is that rationality is not an ideal state to which we aspire, but imperfectly realize, instead it is a capacity which is integral to feeling, needing creatures like us. Preferring the intuitive to the rational life is not an option. As Kant pointed out, the dove flying through the air feeling its resistance, might feel that it could fly so much more freely if there were no air at all. Similarly, when we encounter difficulties in reasoning, it may be tempting to think that life would be easier if we abandoned reason. In reality there is no other *human* way of life to take its place. While we can be, and most of us often are, irrational, what we cannot be is non-rational. We are obliged to drive rationality as far we can. There are, and must be, some areas where belief alone must suffice. But just as it is a mistake to forget this and produce an overrationalistic view of life, so it is a mistake to have recourse to this truth too early and to forget the fundamental role of argument.

Further reading

Beginner

Emmet, E.R. 1964: *Learning to philosophize*. Harmondsworth: Pelican.
Hodges, W. 1977: *Logic*. Harmondsworth: Penguin.
Passmore, J. 1961: *Philosophical reasoning*. London: Duckworth.

Intermediary

Lemmon, E.J. 1965: *Beginning logic*. London: Nelson University Paperbacks.
Salmon, W.C. 1963: *Logic*. Englewood Cliffs, NJ.: Prentice-Hall.

Advanced

Quine, W.V. 1952: *Methods of logic*. London: Routledge and Kegan Paul.
Strawson, P.F. 1952: *Introduction to logical theory*. London: Methuen.

Philosophy of knowledge

Introduction

Nursing is very much a practical discipline. Whatever the speciality of the nurse, her or his role will involve doing things which have an impact on the lives of others in very immediate ways. This doing may involve physical activities, such as bathing patients, or less physically active forms of care, such as counselling, but it will always involve practical activity. This activity, however, also involves an intellectual element – the planning, decision-making, organizing and evaluation of practice – and without this element, nursing care can become dangerously thoughtless.

It has been common in nursing, and in philosophy, to regard the areas of thinking and doing as separate types of activity, which are hopefully related, but essentially different. This separation, which is sometimes referred to as 'dualism' or the mind–body divide, is reflected in the way in which nursing curricula are written, which separately discusses learning experiences as classroom or practical sessions, and in many of the debates about the best way in which to develop nursing knowledge.

To crudely simplify the two main stances taken in this debate, we can see these stances as emphasizing either thinking or doing as the source and focus of nursing knowledge. On the 'doing' side, we have the argument that intellectual reflection is worthless if nurses cannot carry out the caring activities which patients clearly require. The spectre is raised of the intellectual nurse, faced with an emergency, say a patient bleeding profusely from a wound, who discourses knowledgeably on the mechanisms of blood clotting, while the patient dies because she has not applied a tourniquet.

On the 'thinking' side we have the spectre of the nurse unthinkingly carrying out procedures in absolute ignorance of the principles behind her actions. Patients are starved before surgery, regardless of the time of their operation, because routine rather than understanding dictates. As a consequence, they can go to theatre suffering from malnutrition. Slavish following of practice routines results in patients' pressure sores being painted with all kinds of potions which not only fail to promote healing, but are also dangerous. Simply doing, argue the thinking camp, is not enough: there needs to be some intellectual understanding of care.

Both sides, of course, have a point. Nursing is not simply the mindless carrying out of physical duties, nor is it merely an academic reflection on the phenomena of illness. What is interesting, however, is that these two positions ever came to exist, and that it has taken so long for nursing to attempt to reconcile them. Perhaps this debate needs to be seen in a wider context, which involves not only the parallel debates in philosophy but their impact on the way in which knowledge is defined and evaluated throughout society. The debate in philosophy about what sorts of things can be counted as knowledge and further hierarchical arrangements of knowledge into different categories has tended to encourage the view that not only can knowledge be identified and classified, but also that what remains outside these boundaries can be referred to as ignorance. As no professional group wants to be accused of ignorance (after all, being called a 'profession' is partly based on the possession of a recognized body of knowledge), it is dangerous to stray too far from accepted definitions of knowledge.

Dunlop (1986) made this point well when she described the tendency in nursing to overemphasize the intellectual credentials of nursing at the expense of publicizing the tasks that nurses do. She argued that, because these tasks involve things which are distasteful or taboo to many, there has been a move towards focusing on the 'cleaner' aspects of nursing – the body becomes more ethereal, and nursing becomes disembodied. This observation fits, to some extent, with those who feel that the emphasis on academic nursing is largely driven by a desire to gain social status for the profession.

Emphasizing the academic side of nursing, however, would not raise the status of the profession if academic thought was not generally held in high regard throughout the rest of society. To understand why it is, however, we need to trace through the debates about knowledge which have occurred in philosophy and their impact on general thinking and values. This chapter discusses this, and also presents some of the more recent anti-dualist thought which has developed this century, in the attempt to come to some way of reconciling intellectual and anti-intellectual positions in nursing.

Knowledge theory

The fundamental problem for the theory of knowledge is distinguishing between knowledge and belief, between being able to claim to know something about the world and merely claiming to believe something about the world. Why does this contrast matter? Why devote so much energy to worrying about the distinction?

The classical answer to this question is that to claim to know something is a much stronger claim than to believe it. When I say that I believe something, what am I claiming? I seem to be reporting a psychological fact about myself, namely that I take something to be the case, to be true. For example, let us say that I claim to believe that Prozac has harmful side-effects and my claim is sincere. What this means is that I take it to be the case that this drug has harmful side-effects. My being in this psychological state has implications for my behaviour. Thus I am perhaps less likely to use the drug myself, to recommend it to others, and so on. I hold something in the world to be the case, that Prozac is harmful and I hold a particular statement to be true, the statement that 'Prozac has harmful side-effects'.

Now, what happens if a major research trial finds conclusively that Prozac does not, in fact, have harmful side-effects whatsoever, but on the contrary is entirely benign? Will I now say that I never really believed it anyway? Well, I may, if I am dishonest or self-deceiving. But if I am truthful, I will say that, though I used to believe Prozac to have harmful side-effects, the belief that I had was false. I believed it all right but I was wrong. What this means is that beliefs, which form some of my psychological states, can be true or false. This sounds perfectly obvious, indeed trivial.

The point of this obvious sounding remark, however, becomes apparent when we take the case of knowledge. Imagine now that I claim to know that Prozac has harmful side-effects. Again, I am disposed not to recommend it, to avoid its use and so on. And again, a major research trial finds conclusively that Prozac does not, in fact, have harmful side-effects. What can I say now? Can I say that though I knew it, my knowledge was in fact false? No. This is nonsense. It does not make sense to say, 'I falsely knew that something was the case' whereas it did make sense to say that 'I falsely believed that something was the case'.

What this means is that for anything P, it is a condition of my knowing P that P really is true, whereas it is not a condition of my believing P, that P really be true. I might believe P but P might be false. It follows that when I claim to know something I am doing something more that just reporting something about my psychological states.

Of course, knowing something does involve being in a particular psychological state. In particular, it involves believing something! The truth of this strange remark becomes apparent when we try to imagine someone saying, 'Oh yes, I know that Prozac has harmful side-effects but I don't believe it'. What might someone mean by this odd remark? Perhaps that though they knew that Prozac was not wholly a good thing, they were still astonished at the fact (perhaps they been taking it a long time in preference to a drug that had been known for a long time to have bad effects). But this interpretation aside, this remark does not make sense. If someone knows something, then they certainly believe it. What this means is that when I claim to know something, I believe it to be true and, quite independently of my belief, it really is true. If this were the end of the story about knowledge then we could simply say that knowledge consists in having true beliefs.

But is it the end of the story? Imagine the following case. Smith goes along to his village fête and enters the 'Guess the number of beans in the jar' competition. She takes one look at the jar and says '33609'. When the beans are counted, it turns out that Smith is not just the nearest to the right number but has got the number exactly right. Now, Smith certainly has a true belief about the number of beans in the jar, namely that there were 33609 of them. But would any of us claim that Smith knew the number of beans in the jar when she made her competition entry?

Some of us may say, 'Well, if she got it exactly right, she must have known!' And this means something like 'she cheated, it wasn't a fair competition' and so on. But what if we exclude cheating as a possibility? Most of us will say that she did not – could not – have known the number of beans. She just made a lucky guess. But if this is right, there must be more to knowledge than just having true beliefs for Smith certainly has a true belief about the number of beans but she did not know it.

To take an example from nursing; if Nurse Jones believes an unconscious patient admitted to an emergency room to have diabetes, which is later confirmed by the results of tests, then can we say that Nurse Jones 'knew' that this was the case? There were many other conditions that the patient may have had, and given the lack of information available to Nurse Jones, any of them would have been equally likely.

What then is missing from the analysis of knowledge as true belief? It will strike most of us that what is missing is an account of how Smith or Jones came to acquire their (admitted) true beliefs. What reasons did they have for believing what they did? What justification did they have? Imagine that Smith was able to tell some complicated story about how the light bounced off the jar and how she was able to make a calculation based upon this. We should be amazed that there is such a method but we would now be quite happy to say that she did know the number of beans after all. Similarly, if Jones argued that she knew the patient had diabetes because of the particular smell of his breath, then her knowledge would become more justified.

What this means then is that knowledge is, at least, justified true belief. And this is the classical picture of the nature of knowledge. Why does this matter? Because now, when we claim to know something we are claiming that there is some reason for our belief, some evidence we can point to, some methodology we followed: and these are reasons, evidence and methodologies that can be shared by others. Beliefs are essentially private psychological facts. But knowledge is, in principle, public and sharable. Therefore, when we claim to know something, we are doing more than just making a claim about ourselves and more than just making a claim about the world. Implicitly, we are making a claim that what we know about is amenable to rational, and perhaps systematic, investigation.

One job of the theory of knowledge has been to try and spell what justification must mean in this context. Exactly what counts as justification and what does not? Within philosophy, there have been radical disagreements about the sources of justifications for knowledge claims. Indeed, such disputes have shaped much of the history of philosophy. In what follows we describe the outlines of this dispute.

Rationalist theories of knowledge

Sophists

It is not surprising that early Greek philosophers were very much concerned with examining the notion of knowledge – what it is possible to know, what can be known for certain and how knowledge can be challenged. Such questions are fundamental to philosophy and particularly so when philosophy was beginning to be mapped out – there needed to be some guidelines for developing such a map. It is also not surprising that early Greek ideas of knowledge were essentially rationalist, in other words that they were predicated on the belief that valid knowledge could, and should, be achieved by the exercise of reason alone; empirical science was in its infancy and had yet to achieve the prominence that it did later.

One of the earliest theories of knowledge was that propounded by the Sophists who argued that it was extremely doubtful that anything could be known with great certainty, and therefore it was useless to strive after something which was unobtainable. The only way to evaluate or judge knowledge was at an individual level, according to that individual's nature and requirements – 'Man is the measure of all things'. This position is a powerful one, and it is possible to trace its influence throughout the following centuries of intellectual debate, but sophistry has also been regarded with great suspicion by many; indeed, to be accused of sophistry is to be accused of intellectual evasiveness. This is because the Sophists, after making their basic assertion, did not spend too much time in building up a careful analysis of the ways in which individual judgement of knowledge could operate, but instead moved to a position in which they focused on the skills required to win debates. Since all knowledge was uncertain, it was useless to examine it and therefore debates would be won on the strength of debating skills. Sophists, therefore, concentrated on teaching their followers how to argue persuasively to support their position, rather than to examine that position.

Plato and Socrates

The argument that all knowledge is relative to the person of the knower, and that debates should not centre on a striving for the truth was anathema to later Greek philosophers who were attempting to find some certainty in their world, or at least examine ways in which this could be achieved. The notion of sophists winning arguments and influence by successfully arguing positions which they themselves did not accept, was a dangerous one especially if (as in the work of Plato) a system of philosophy was being aspired to which would form the basis for ordering all aspects of life and human enquiry. For Plato, there were some things which remained constant and unchanging rather than relative, and it was in the apprehension of these things ('ideas' or 'forms' as Plato called them) that true knowledge lay. The constancy of forms prevailed regardless of our direct experience of them – indeed, our experiences of forms is only through examples of them. For example, we could point to several different horses, of varying shapes and sizes, and reasonably call them all 'horses'. This general term is used to classify creatures which are visibly quite different, but it makes sense to do this because we have some idea of what the general term means. As to how we know what general terms or forms mean, Plato referred to Socrates' argument that knowledge cannot be learnt, but only recollected. In other words, that we are born with knowledge of forms, rather than taught them, and the job of philosophy is to help us recollect and rediscover them. Socrates gives the example of an uneducated slave boy who is asked to calculate the area of a square. By criticizing his responses, rather than telling him how to do the calculation, Socrates leads him to the correct answer, and concludes that if the boy can do this without education or instruction, then he must have already, in some way, known the answer.

The type of knowledge which deals with Platonic ideas, the abstract definitions of universal forms, is also contrasted with knowledge acquired through the senses – 'sensible knowledge'. Socrates argued that sensible knowledge is a shadowy and blurred type of knowledge and open to distortion, and he illustrates this point by using the example of men imprisoned in a cave where they can only see the shadows of their captors. If they only had the evidence of their senses, their conception of their captors would be very strange, and they would need to use rational knowledge to understand the true nature of those who held them prisoner. The allegory of the cave was more than a demonstration of the unreliability of the senses, however, as Socrates talked about what would happen if the prisoners were brought out into the sun. They would initially be blinded by the light, but would eventually recover and appreciate their new-found clarity of sight. Socrates used this allegory, not as an illustration of how sensory information could be improved, but as an illustration of how people could leave the 'prison of the senses' and achieve true knowledge through entering the intellectual plane.

This journey to the intellectual world, Socrates asserted, could be achieved by following a system of instruction, which would first start off with a recognition of the vagaries of sense information. From there, the student would progress through the study of arithmetic, geometry, astronomy and harmonics (the study of sound) until ready for the dialectic – the examining of assumptions and definitions and the consequent understanding of Platonic ideas. Mathematics and the other studies would prepare the student for this by introducing the notion of abstract forms, and then the student would be able to examine forms and universals without reference to the sensory world of appearances.

Descartes

The mistrust of sensory knowledge exhibited by Socrates and Plato was echoed some centuries later by the seventeenth century philosopher Descartes. Descartes was a philosopher, natural scientist and mathematician at a time when such disciplines were not separated in the way that they are now. Believing that mathematics was the foundation of natural science, in that mathematics could form a means of expressing the relationships that natural science discovered, he went further and argued that mathematics provided a paradigm of certain knowledge.

Descartes' method, then, was to apply to all assertions of belief a 'test', that is he would examine them according to whether they met his criteria of being 'clearly and distinctly true'. By this he meant that they would be intrinsically true in the same way as mathematical and logical propositions would be true – if any doubt could be entertained, or any other possible explanations could be admitted, then the assertions would be rejected. What was left over at the end of this process would be certain knowledge.

Examining things known to him through his senses, he was immediately aware that these could be doubted. Physical objects looked and felt real, but he reasoned that he had often experienced them in such a way when he had been dreaming – when they were not real. As there was no way to distinguish between an object experienced when awake and that in a dream, he concluded that the physical world experienced through the senses, even his own body, was open to doubt. The only thing that could not be doubted was the fact that he was doubting, in other words that he was able to reason and think. It was the only proof that he existed even if all else was potentially illusory, and could not be open to doubt, as the process of doubting is, by definition, evidence of thinking. Furthermore, thinking was proof of existence – it does not make sense to assert that something can think without existing, and this idea was expressed in the famous Cartesian formula *Cogito ergo sum* or 'I am thinking, therefore I exist'.

Descartes' use of the term 'thinking' is not necessarily restricted to intellectual analysis – he recognized the existence of other types of cognitive processes. The experience of objects was such a phenomenon – to have such an experience was to think of such objects as if they were there. In this sense, the objects must exist in some way, if only in his thoughts. Extending this observation to other things that he thinks exist, he finds that one of the things that he thinks of is the idea of God. God does not exist, however, only as something in his mind, in the way that a table or chair might, but must be external to his mind – it is not possible for an imperfect being, such as Descartes, to create in his mind something which is perfect. So the fact that he thinks of God proves that God exists.

Having established the existence of God through this line of reasoning, Descartes returns to his notion of illusory objects. He argues that a perfect being, God, would not allow him to be so deceived, and would not allow him to believe in things which did not exist. It follows, then, that the world of objects is real, but we must be suspicious of it and critical of our impressions. This rather circular argument allows Descartes to believe in the world as a product of God – a fortunate conclusion since it therefore enabled him to treat food and drink and other things necessary to the continuation of his corporeal existence as real.

Descartes did not, therefore, starve himself to death believing that hunger was illusory, partly because of his reference to God, but also because he treated the body as a special type of object. It was not completely separate from the mind, given that it enabled the mind to experience the world, but it was not the same type of thing as the mind. The exact nature of the relationship between the body and the mind was one which, he felt, was ultimately unexplainable, although he did make some attempts to do so. These attempts centred on his avowal of dualism, that there were two types of substance 'souls' and matter, or thinking and extended substances. While matter or extended substance was subject to the laws of natural science, the soul would remain outside these laws. Though linked, soul and matter were distinct from each other, and to this degree were separate.

Empiricism

From the summary of some of the work of the rationalist philosophers given above, it can be seen that there are two characteristics of their position, namely the distrust of sensory experience as a source of knowledge, and an anti-relativist stance which leads to the search for certainty. Both of these elements were challenged by a group of philosophers usually called the empiricists. This term is used because it describes their chief concern, the nature of the knowledge gained from sensory experience of the world. This concern arises from the limitations of rationalism. If rationalist philosophies can be shown to incorporate arguments which are not derived from pure reason then their claims to superior methodology are suspect. Furthermore, their insistence on treating the everyday world of experience as insubstantial, or a source of error, seems to ignore a major part of human existence, and raises questions about the purpose of this philosophy – how can it improve life in a domain it rejects? The search for certainty rests upon the assumption that such certainty exists, and some empiricists would argue that this is an unwarranted assumption. The fact that people can live their lives without such certainty has suggested to some empiricists that efforts would be better spent on finding out how this is done rather than simply dismissing it as an irrational phenomenon outside the scope of philosophy.

Empiricism developed most vigorously in places and periods when the natural world began to be understood more, and this knowledge harnessed in the development of technology. Given the achievements of scientists such as Isaac Newton or Robert Boyle, it became difficult to maintain that such scientific endeavour dealt only with shadows, and as these discoveries informed technology, and therefore industry and commerce, and had a great impact on everyday life, it became important to try to explain how these discoveries were possible.

Locke

Locke was one of the foremost thinkers in empirical philosophy, who in the latter half of the seventeenth century, began to argue that knowledge came to us through our senses and our observation and experience of the physical world, rather than, as Socrates had asserted, we are born with knowledge. Locke argued that we acquire knowledge; his aim then becomes to analyse this process of acquisition – to tell us what we can know, and what sort of certainty we can have.

Locke asserted that we have two ways of knowing things: by sensation and by reflection. Through these two modes we receive impression of an object's primary or secondary qualities – primary qualities being things such as size and shape which belong to the things themselves, and secondary qualities being things such as colours, which are the product of powers in the object to produce, in certain conditions, certain sensations in our minds. The distinction Locke makes here is between the scientific reporting of objects (concerned with primary qualities) and the everyday experience of those objects (secondary qualities). The qualities of the objects that we perceive lead us to develop 'simple ideas', i.e. those not compounded of other elements, such as the sweetness of sugar or the smell of a rose. These ideas are observed to occur in combinations in a consistent way; gold, for example, will combine the ideas of hardness, colour and lustre. We therefore presume that these ideas belong to something.

From our experience of simple ideas we can begin to develop knowledge, and Locke identified four ways in which this can be done. Firstly, we can compare ideas to see if they are the same or different. Secondly, we can see if ideas occur or belong together. Thirdly, we can see if ideas are related together. Fourthly, we can see if ideas exist outside of our minds or not, in other words whether they are ideas of real existences. These questions that we ask about our ideas, Locke argues, are all that we can know.

There are different types of certainty that we can have about these types of knowledge. Firstly, we can know intuitively that things are the case – we immediately know that they are true, 'the mind is presently filled with the clear light of it'. Secondly, we can know things are true through demonstration – step-by-step reasoning, or as Locke argued, a series of linked intuitions. Demonstration, however, can never be as sure as intuition alone as we may miss out steps along the way. Thirdly, we can achieve some degree of certainty through sensitive knowledge, which can at least assure us, to all practical purposes, that things exist. Sensitive knowledge, however, is subject to the inconsistencies and problems of all sensory experiences. At this point, Locke's argument seems to suggest that the most important knowledge of all – that things do exist – is dependent on the least sure form of certainty, which he argues is sensitive knowledge. Thus Locke comes dangerously close to the distrust of the senses displayed by the rationalists.

Locke's way out of the position that knowledge of objects is simply subjective mental impressions, is that our knowledge is, ultimately, not simply our imagination. The building up of simple ideas must be a reflection of reality, because it is not possible to construct these out of nothing – they have no constituent elements. Nevertheless, Locke's thesis reveals the central problem of empiricism, which is that any theory of knowledge which sees that knowledge as coming from outside us, through our senses, must acknowledge the vagaries of those senses. If the empiricists do not reject sensory knowledge as the rationalists do, as being illusory, they must come up with some firm basis for accepting it. Locke's work, although intending to provide such a basis, does not do so, partly because in his system of knowledge perception of things is still distinguished from the existence of things. He still distinguishes between things as they are and things as we experience them, and by making this initial distinction, creates problems for himself as he tries to find ways round it.

Berkeley

Other empiricists, for example Bishop Berkeley, have identified this problem. Berkeley argued that as soon as we cast doubts on the reliability of our sensory information 'we are insensibly drawn into uncouth paradoxes, difficulties and inconsistencies, which multiply and grow upon us as we advance in speculation; till at length, having wandered through many intricate mazes, we find ourselves just where we were or, which is worse, sit down in forlorn scepticism'. This type of venture leads philosophy into disrepute and makes its debates a matter of amusement for non-philosophers, and eventually, Berkeley argues will lead ordinary people to doubt the existence of God.

One of Berkeley's main objections to Locke's theory was his distinction between primary and secondary qualities, and his suggestion that the former are 'real' whereas the latter are illusory. There are no grounds for making this distinction, Berkeley argues, and the distinction is empirically inconsistent – all sensory information should be treated in the same way. Berkeley's thesis, which asserts that all knowledge is essentially empirical, places emphasis on sensation and perception, leading to the conclusion that things only exist if they are perceived – that objects do not exist outside this perception. Berkeley then proposed a theory of immaterialism. He argued that since all we can perceive is an idea, which must exist in a mind, and that we cannot control these ideas, they must belong to some other mind – the mind of God. As God's mind is universal and permanent, then when things are not in a person's mind, they are still in God's.

Berkeley's immaterialism was greeted with great cynicism and ridicule by his contemporaries. His emphasis on things as only being ideas seemed to suggest that the world was an insubstantial dream. In this he echoed some rationalist thought, and did not achieve his aim of producing a thesis which corresponded with the outlook of ordinary people.

Hume

Berkeley's difficulties in producing a theory of knowledge which corresponded with the experience of everyday knowledge were felt by Hume to arise mainly from his failure to start with an examination of how ordinary people thought. Hume's work, therefore, began with this ordinary thinking, and he believed that if we could understand more about human nature, then we could understand more about how knowledge is developed. In this way,

Hume's work resembles what we would now call psychology rather than the excessively abstract philosophical tradition which had, until then, prevailed.

Hume argued that everything that we are aware of can be classified as either impressions or ideas, which differ according to the force with which they 'strike upon the mind', with impressions being more forceful than ideas. Ideas and impressions can be simple or complex, but on examination, Hume argued, we find that complex ideas cannot be traced back to complex impressions, as impressions are invariably simple. We then can build simple impressions into complex ideas. We are aided in this process by our ability to use the faculties of memory and imagination.

Memory is especially important, as it means that we can have a series of ideas in our heads which are in fixed order or sequence, and we can link ideas together. This association of ideas, Hume argued, suggests a kind of attraction between them, analogous to the types of attraction which were at that time being suggested in the natural world. This attraction, however, can be misleading, Hume stated, as it can lead us to assume a causality which may be erroneous. If we link ideas together, by observing or remembering a pattern of succession or contiguity between them, we go a step further and presume some sort of causal link between them. This link, however, does not come from any impression or anything that we observe, or from any feature of the two ideas or impression, and thus represents an idea which does not come directly from our experience – it is, rather, something which arises from our interpretation of experience.

Hume then went on to examine this notion of causality in more depth, and in particular the assumption that everything must have a cause. This cannot be proved by scientific or logical reasoning, since these arguments, in Hume's analysis, presuppose causality from the start. The idea of causality, therefore must come from our experience in some way (assuming that we are not born with an innate knowledge of it, as Socrates would argue). Our idea of causality, Hume argued, arises from our experience in the way that we can remember patterns of ideas. Hume pointed out that we experience certain ideas or impressions in constant conjunction; for example we bite into an apple and experience a particular taste. We can then experience only one of these impressions, say the sight of an apple, and from the past we will remember the taste and will expect it to be the same. This expectation, Hume points out, rests on the assumption that the world is uniform. Without this assumption, there is no reason to expect that biting into an apple will cause a particular taste sensation – it may well cause something else, say, the taste of fish. It is always possible that the world may turn topsy-turvy overnight, and that fire will feel cold, or snow will feel hot, but we presume that the uniformity that we experience today will persist. The principle of uniformity, then, is fundamental to the way in which we know the world, a mysterious belief which Hume attributed to psychological habit brought about by the forcefulness of our ideas and impressions, and of the patterns in which they occur.

This quirk of human nature, which leads us to expect, without any logical or possible proof, that the world is uniform, leads us also to expect that experiences which we have not had will resemble experiences that we have had. It is therefore a feature of human nature, or psychology, and is fundamental to understanding the type of knowledge which we feel we have. It is not a feature of the things that we experience – there is nothing about the sight of an apple which tells us of its taste.

The consequence of Hume's deliberations was that knowledge, as human beings have it, depends not only upon experience, but on the mind which interprets it. This interpretation, Hume argued from a sceptical position, was not supported by any empirical evidence, but was rather based on beliefs which originated in the peculiar psychology of human beings. He then concluded that most of what we call 'knowledge' is really a matter of belief, and therefore subject to the vagaries of the person holding such beliefs. Under examination, even our philosophical debates and positions could be seen to be more a matter of preference and psychological quirks rather than anything else.

Modern theories

The dilemmas posed by the rationalist–empiricist debate are broadly as follows. If the search for certain knowledge is seen as being achieved by the exercise of reason, the experienced world becomes doubtful to the extent that rationalist theories bear little resemblance to the everyday development of knowledge. If knowledge is seen as being derived from experience, it becomes difficult to account for things that we think we know which are not directly experienced.

These problems arise partly from the concentration of the philosophers involved on the nature of knowledge in some 'pure' form, and so it is not surprising that the most recent work in this field has turned its attention to the way in which knowledge is applied and used. This work has, as Hume claimed to have, a basis in the everyday exercise of knowledge – the practical aspects.

Pragmatism

Some of the most important work in this century has come from a group of philosophers not surprisingly called the pragmatists, who include John Dewey and William James. The pragmatists originated in America at a time when the old metaphysical philosophy was felt to have run out of steam. In a country which was intent on developing a new identity and moving away from its cultural roots in Europe, such a move in philosophy echoed general developments in American culture.

Their emphasis is on problem-solving – they argued that the purpose of philosophy was to solve intellectual problems rather than simply create or define them, as had been the emphasis in European philosophy, and this ethos was reflected in their theories of knowledge. One essential feature of pragmatism was that the test of any theory was to see what its consequences were, what difference it would make if it were true or false. If it made no difference whatsoever to the way that people thought or lived, then it was a worthless theory. This emphasis on the utility of philosophy is evident in pragmatist theories of knowledge: there is a concern with the way in which knowledge is used.

Dewey was particularly influential in his theories of knowledge, and developed a view which came to be known as instrumentalism, largely because it was concerned with the way in which knowledge was used. According to Dewey, we have experiences which are essentially the interactions between a biological organism and the environment in which it lives. Experience then, is not the rather passive 'being struck' by impressions or objects, but it is about performing actions. When an organism meets situations in which it cannot act, then thinking occurs as a means of dealing with these situations. The criteria by which such thought should be judged concerns the degree to which this thinking allows the organism to act. His famous comment 'the True is that which works' illustrates the way in which he replaced the problem of truth, which had occupied the classical philosophers, with that of utility.

Dewey's instrumentalism has had a great impact on educational methods, as one would expect from a philosophy which emphasizes the practical. He argued that much of education was concerned with the memorizing of factual information, whereas the central focus should be on equipping students to solve problems. His philosophy led to what was called 'progressive education' where students would be confronted with questions and problems to solve. There are variants of this approach to be found in nurse education today: the work of Schon, for example, with his discussion of the practicum, in which the world of practice would be replicated and students coached through problem-solving, has become extremely popular.

There are, however, some difficulties with Dewey's philosophy. The most important is that which arises when we consider what we would mean when we said that something 'worked'. Dewey's response would be essentially that something works if it allows us to act, but acting alone cannot be a determinant of utility – we would want to distinguish between acting well and acting badly. Utility of thinking is therefore linked to the value of this thinking in the way that it achieves desired aims (themselves the product of values). A further problem was identified by Russell, who argued that for a theory to work, it must in some way correspond with reality. Theories, then, cannot simply be judged by their utility – they must also be true by correspondence. Knowledge, then, is not simply a human construction, but must take into account things as they are, otherwise it will fail the test of utility.

Existentialism

Another modern approach to knowledge has been developed by a group of philosophers now called existentialists. This grouping is not necessarily one that they themselves would have approved of, given that they had many differences of opinion, but it is a term which usefully conveys their main concern – to understand the nature of human existence. Their concern was not, therefore, expressly with the problem of knowledge, but much of what they wrote has some bearing on it. By exploring how people exist, they also explore the nature of the relationship between people and the world that they exist in and respond to. This response is largely determined by the way in which they know about the world.

The existential concern is, broadly speaking, to understand people in the way that they exist 'in the world', that is not as something separate from the world but as beings which are rooted in the everyday life. In addition to this broad interest, the existentialists are also concerned with the notion of people as 'free' in that they make choices about how they live. This anti-deterministic stance therefore directs existentialist philosophy to a study of how people can be shown to be free, and the nature of the choices that they can make. These related concerns, about the nature of human existence, and the freedoms that it involves, require an approach to philosophical enquiry which addresses directly the phenomena of human life which is rooted in these phenomena, rather than in the more abstract debate evident in other philosophical traditions.

This phenomenological enquiry is usually held to have originated in the work of Husserl, although it has gone through several changes and revisions since. Husserl's phenomenology was essentially a 'scientific' method, in that he viewed the phenomenologist as one who would study human phenomena in the same way that non-human phenomena are studied, from a detached, rather than emotionally involved stance. These human phenomena were what would now be called 'psychology', the feelings, thoughts and emotions, and their study was, for Husserl, to be achieved by the description of the immediate experiences or perceptions of the objects which give rise to these feelings, or to which they are directed to. This directedness, or intentionality was, for Husserl, the crucial characteristic of human thinking, that thoughts are always directed to objects. The study of thoughts is descriptive in the sense that all assumptions or ideas about how things are experienced or perceived (or indeed about the things themselves) must be suspended, and the concern is on faithfully recording the experiences themselves.

Husserl's phenomenology thus turns thoughts into objects, and as such echoed some of the psychological aspects of Hume's philosophy. In some ways he also followed the Cartesian tradition of dualism, in his assertion that intellectual enquiry was distinct from experience of the world and as such displays many of the problems associated with this position. By separating experience from analysis of that experience, divisions arise between the intellectual and the physical – a division that other existentialists sought to break down.

Heidegger, in particular, reacted against this subject–object division and against the notion of directedness or intentionality. He questioned the notion that our experience of things was always subjective (in the sense that we are always subjects) and illustrated this point by identifying situations in which people would engage with the world without the subject–object relationship. One example which Heidegger gave was that of the expert carpenter, who uses a hammer without thinking about it in any conscious way at all – the hammer is transparent to him. Heidegger argued that much of human contact with the world is of this nature, and that the relationship is not always that of a conscious subject directed towards an independent object.

Heidegger's argument suggests that people are primarily in and of the world, rather than subjects in a world of objects. This situation Heidegger refers to as *Dasein*, a term which can be translated as 'being there' ('there' can be taken as 'the world' and thus an alternative interpretation is perhaps the more evocative 'being in the world'). Being human is, therefore, a situated activity, a situation in which things are encountered and managed.

The notion of *Dasein* contains three different elements. Firstly, there is the element of attunement or mood. Because of this, things matter. Secondly, there is the element of discourse or articulation, whereby things are related to their function. Returning to the example of the hammer, it can be articulated as a hammer by hammering with it. Thirdly, there is the element of managing the world in order to achieve a goal – the 'for the sake of' our activities. These three elements of *Dasein* represent the past, present and future of a person; attunement is the way in which we meet experience, articulation is the way in which we have experience and goals are where our experience leads us – our potential.

The central problem of this being for the existentialist project of freedom, however, is that it can become forgotten. Because people are so immersed in the world and so adept at living in it, they do not think of it as something which needs any further enquiry. Because of this 'taking for granted' of the world, the potential and choices of human beings can become forgotten. This then, is the purpose of Heidegger's phenomenology, which he called 'hermeneutic', to reveal the significance and nature of the world.

Hermeneutics, however, has inherent problems. How are we to interpret our experience, or to have any measure of the validity of our interpretations? There is a feeling that by stressing the subjectivity of interpretation, the existentialists have adopted an extremely relativist stance, and the quest for truth and certainty has been abandoned. Like Dewey's pragmatism, existentialism seems to be arguing that truth is determined by context and also by person.

Nursing knowledge

We can now return to the debate that we began with – what is the nature of knowledge and furthermore, how can it be evaluated? We have seen how the rationalists sought to describe knowledge, and how their quest for certainty led them to see the experiential world as a source of confusion. We have also seen how the empiricists sought to describe how knowledge can be derived from experience, but how their failure to describe differences between knowledge and the world of objects led them to either fall into rationalism or to conclude that knowledge is relative, or determined by the psychology of the individual. By focusing on the way knowledge is used, rather than on what it is, modern theorists have avoided some of these problems, but have created another, namely how we can judge the use of knowledge. It is with these debates in mind that we return to the issues that were outlined at the beginning of this chapter – how we can think about nursing knowledge.

To return to the point made at the beginning of this chapter, nursing is essentially a practical discipline. As such it deals with the physical world, which it cannot regard as illusory. Regarding the bodies of nurses and patients as mere figments of our imagination, does not help people to health; indeed, it calls the whole venture into question. Accepting that our work deals in the world of experience, and has a vital empirical base, however, still leads us to the problem of how we assess and evaluate that base. We can probably all think of times when our senses deceived us, and there is enough literature on psychosomatic disorders to indicate that the senses of our patients also can deceive them.

What do we do about these delusions? One way in which we deal with the evidence of our senses is to make it public and open to scrutiny. We use measuring instruments that can be used by others, we record our observations so that others can confirm or question them. In cases where there is agreement, we can at least say that the evidence of senses seems to be the same for everyone, and on that basis we can proceed. We cannot, however, regard this sensory knowledge as anything more than provisional – someone may come along who has a very different experience or who interprets that experience differently. Where there is disagreement we tend to be more explicit about the provisional nature of knowledge, we talk of competing interpretations, and following these through, looking at the implications of them in terms of the action that they suggest. The action that we take is based on our assessments of the risks involved in being right or wrong. If interpretation X suggests action A, and interpretation Y suggests action B, we will tend to opt for the interpretation which leads to the lower risk if we are wrong – the risks involved in taking action A or B. Interestingly, our way of dealing with the sensory delusions of patients is either to dismiss them or to treat them as 'real' enough to warrant psychiatric help.

This suggests a degree of pragmatism – what is true is what works (or at least is not likely to fail disastrously). Our pragmatism, however, tends to take for granted our ideas of what 'works'. To take an example, many years ago it was common for terminally ill patients to be given limited analgesia because it was 'addictive'. It took the hospice movement to suggest that what works in this situation is relieving pain rather than preventing addiction. Nursing knowledge therefore must not only be provisional, but must regard its values as provisional too.

The existential view of knowledge also has implications for nursing. The description that Heidegger gives of a carpenter and his tools, which are used without conscious awareness, reflects many situations in nursing in which action takes place at some sort of intuitive or automatic level. This sort of knowledge, however, comes with familiarity and experience, as researchers like Benner have pointed out. A novice nurse or carpenter is unable to operate in this way, the tools feel uncomfortable, or as Heidegger might put it, they are operating as a subject in a world of objects, they are not yet 'in the world'.

The implications for nurse education are several. Firstly, nurses need to be aware of the provisional nature of the knowledge that they derive from the senses, and training a nurse must involve teaching them ways of confirming or disputing this knowledge, and of making their processes of acquisition public. Secondly, the element of pragmatism, and the values on which ideas of 'working' are based must be made more explicit and open to challenge. Thirdly, the existential aspects of knowledge need to be fostered, in that nurses need to have the practical experience necessary for them to become part of the world of nursing.

This analysis suggests that nursing knowledge must be both theoretical and practical, and that neither alone will suffice. Identifying two types of knowledge still looks like a continuation of dualism, but there is a difference between earlier conceptions, in that one is not privileged to the exclusion of the other. Using the idea of all knowledge as provisional, and certainty as relative allows us to reformulate the relationship between practical and theoretical knowledge in a different way – as counterbalancing and contributing to each other. Practical knowledge can act as a check against theory, and theory can act as a check against practice. The development of nursing knowledge, therefore depends on making this relationship clearer and more explicit.

References

Dunlop, M.J. 1986: Is a science of caring possible? *Journal of Advanced Nursing* **11**, 661–70.

Further reading

Ayer, A.J. 1956: *The problem of knowledge*. Harmondsworth: Penguin.
Berkeley, G. 1975: *Treatise concerning the principles of human knowledge*. London: Dent.
Descartes, R. 1960: *Metaphysical meditations*. Harmondsworth: Penguin.
Dewey, J. 1956: *Reconstruction in philosophy*. London: Muller.
Hume, D. 1975: *An enquiry concerning human understanding*. Oxford: Oxford University Press.
James, W. 1907: In *Pragmatism a new name for some old ways of thinking: popular lectures in philosophy*. New York: Longmans, Green and Co.
Kant, I. 1978: *Critique of judgement*. Oxford: Oxford University Press.
Locke, J. 1964: *An essay concerning human understanding*. London: Collins/Fontana.

Midgely, M. 1989: *Wisdom, information and wonder. What is knowledge for?* London: Routledge.

Vesey, G.N.A. (ed.) 1970: *Knowledge and necessity,* 3. London: Macmillan.

Vesey, G.N.A. (ed.) 1986: *Philosophers ancient and modern*. Royal Institute of Philosophy Lecture Series, 20. Cambridge: Cambridge University Press.

Philosophy of science   4

Introduction

As nursing has developed a more holistic approach to care, attempting to incorporate social and psychological as well as physiological aspects of health and illness into practice, it has necessarily had to widen the scope of its research base. Whereas early research in nursing had followed the traditions of orthodox science developed in the fields of biology and physiology, later research began to broaden out to incorporate social sciences research where there were a number of different ways of viewing science. The strongest challenges to orthodox science came from qualitative researchers who argued that the social world was not appropriately studied in the same way as the physical world and that alternative approaches were needed. This challenge has been supported by many nurse researchers, with the result that nursing research now encompasses a wide range of methodologies and views of science. This plurality of approaches is, arguably, an appropriate route for nursing research to take, but it has created some problems for nursing as an academic discipline. These problems arise from the conflicts and contradictions between the various views of science, which, some would argue, are irreconcilable, and also from the relative status of different views of science within the field of health care (and, most importantly, among those who fund and support health-care research). Nursing, therefore, needs to examine and understand the problems inherent in trying to combine different views of science, and develop a coherent argument to support and explain the combination that it uses. This chapter will be devoted to such an examination, firstly outlining the different positions that are taken on the question of science and its relationship to 'reality', and then going on to discuss the ways in which they can (or cannot) be reconciled. The chapter then moves on to examine some characteristics of nursing practice and their implications for developing ideas about the type of science that is appropriate for nursing.

The bounds of science

In this section we will offer a kind of map of what might be called the 'logical geography' of the philosophy of science, showing the structure of the sorts of questions about scientific endeavour which philosophers have thought it important to ask and to try to answer. The aim is to provide what any philosopher can in the end only offer: greater clarity (though it may be that, as elsewhere in philosophy, the best route to this result is only through greater puzzlement and confusion that one originally started out with).

It would be as well to remove one possible misconception about what we have to say right away. The phrase 'philosophy of science' is not synonymous with 'the general view of the relationship between humans and the universe as derived from the discoveries of modern science', though something at least a little like that does form one aspect of the philosophy of science, and it would be wrong to completely discount it as necessarily too vague and pretentious to be taken seriously. Rather, in general, the philosophy of science is concerned with certain sorts of question that arise about the nature of scientific endeavours in relation to which we are not quite sure as to how to go about finding their answers. That is, the questions which the philosophy of science addresses itself cannot be answered merely by attending closely to the history of science, or to its theories or to what its practitioners have had to say about it, in their more reflective moments. As we shall see, this is because, more often than not, the characteristically philosophical questions that arise about science are concerned with the relationship between science and a whole range of other aspects of human life. Such questions cannot be answered simply by appealing to data because it is the data that force the questions upon us.

We have called this section the 'Bounds of science' because it is with reference to the ambiguities of the word 'bounds' that we want to display the structure of the philosophy of science. We have taken 'bounds' to have three senses: each sense has a corresponding question.

- 'Bounds' in the sense of boundaries
  What are the boundaries of science? The question here is: what, if anything distinguishes science from non-science?
- 'Bounds' in the sense of leaps
  The question here is: what is the explanation, character and consequence of the great revolutions in our understanding of the world that science brings about? In particular, what is the relation between the knowledge that we acquire through science and our ordinary non-scientific beliefs about the world in which we live?
- 'Bounds' in the sense of limits
  The questions here are: are there limits on the competence of science? What sorts of question, if any, is science constitutionally unable to answer?

We will look briefly at each of these areas in turn, to give you some better grip on these questions, their implications and the sorts of answers that have been put forward.

The boundaries of science

Our first question, what, if anything, distinguishes science from non-science, is motivated primarily by the recognition of the enormous success of science over the past 400 years. There is no need here, we are sure, to describe the ways in which scientific endeavour has changed the nature of the human environment, the human world. (A useful exercise here is to choose some especially humble mass-produced object, say adhesive tape, a book of matches or somesuch and to imagine how different our world would have to be if the production of such an object were not in fact possible.) The success of science has been so far reaching in so many directions that in this century, the very term 'scientific' has acquired a commendatory sense: to call some statement 'scientifically proven', no matter what the content of the statement itself, is to appeal to some presumed unique basis of authority which puts the matter beyond dispute. Indeed, for many, the description of one's discipline as science is seen as a precondition of being taken seriously at all. Hence, the preference for 'agricultural science' over 'agriculture' and for the plethora of such disciplines as 'library science', 'administrative science', 'management science' and, in our context, 'nursing science'. The coiners of such terms presumably take themselves to be pointing out something about the nature of their work: that they carry on their work in ways which differ crucially from ways in which such work had been or might be carried out and that they are now likely to be more fruitful than might otherwise have been the case. In short, the presumption is, that in calling their work a 'science', they are applying some method which is both:

- proven to be successful, and
- applicable to their own domain.

The use of the term 'scientific' in this commendatory sense, then, is the invocation of the idea that there is some uniquely successful method of acquiring knowledge which is applicable to domains other than those in which it was first developed. If we take the physical sciences to be the domain in which traditional scientific method developed, then the idea is that these methods are applicable to other domains which are not necessarily about physical phenomena.

It is worth noting here that with the rise of this commendatory sense has come the development of a contrary disapprobatory sense. What is important about this from our point of view is that, while users of these different senses may well be expected to disagree about the value of the knowledge which science has acquired, in the extreme, the one citing X-ray machines and brain scanners, the other thalidomide and nuclear weapons, one frequently finds that they will agree completely about the nature of the method by which this knowledge has been acquired. From both sides we are likely to hear phrases such as 'concerned only with knowledge', 'interested only in facts', 'unemotional', 'not concerned with consequences'. There is, therefore, a fairly detailed conception of the nature of scientific method scientists, among the lay public and critics of science alike.

It is this method which is taken to distinguish science from everything else. In addition, however, it is also thought, though perhaps rather more vaguely, that not every question is answerable through recourse to this method. The traditional image of science in our culture is one defined both by its content, the questions asked, and by its method, the way we go about trying to answer these questions. This can be seen by considering the following question: Which of the following questions and statements do you take to be 'scientific', i.e. admitting of scientific investigation, explanation and answers? (Remember that it is the status, scientific or not, not the truth or falsity, of the statement or answer to the question that is at issue.)

1 This house plant needs to be supported if it is not to die.

2 Most people would prefer this room to be painted white rather than green.

3 *The Tempest* is Shakespeare's last and finest play.

4 Does acupuncture work?

5 Why can't an object be red and green all over its surface?

6 Is fluoride good for teeth?

7 How can we prevent inner-city riots?

8 How far away is the nearest star?

9 This shampoo has been properly tested and is safe to use.

10 $7 + 5 = 12$.

11 Patients with more visitors get well sooner.

12 This patient is ready to leave the hospital.

13 Extra-sensory perception is a real phenomenon.

14 The benefits of research on human embryos would outweigh the risks.

15 Most women prefer female medical staff.

16 Why are there so many different species of living creatures in the world?

17 World War II occurred because of, and not despite, the economic interdependence of European nations.

18 Smoking is bad for your health.

19 How can we improve the longevity of household batteries?

20 Every event has a cause.

21 How did the Universe come into being?

22 It is 75% probable that this person will die of AIDS in the next five years.

23 The next bus will probably be late.

24 Human beings are naturally selfish.

25 Science is the best way of acquiring knowledge about the world.

Now look back through the choices you made and try to decide what criteria you were using to make your choices.

Perhaps you found that you were using something like the following criteria:

- A matter of 'common sense', not science.
- A matter of taste, not a matter of fact.
- A matter of ethics, not a matter of fact.
- A matter of verbal definition, not a matter of fact.
- A matter for literary criticism or history, not science.
- Too particular, not general enough for science.
- Too vague and general, not precise enough for science.
- Advertising hype, not a scientific claim.
- Not interesting enough for science.

The failure to recognize that science is distinguished both by a certain sort of method and by a certain sort of content leads to endless confusion. Thus, someone will claim that the study of the various arts, philosophy and, very often, the social 'sciences' are not at all scientific. If this means that the sorts of questions which these various disciplines ask are not scientific, this is perfectly correct. But because people crudely conflate the sort of questions being asked with the sort of method used to acquire an answer, this is often intended to be some sort of implied criticism: art history is not scientific so not only can its conclusions not be trusted but one person's opinion is as good as anyone else's. For this reason, art history is objectively less important than particle physics.

Now this, of course, is nonsense. The question 'Is this action legal?' is not a scientific question either but it does not follow from this that we cannot have certain answers to it, or that there cannot be experts in it – that it is not a question of knowledge at all and only a matter of opinion.

A parallel confusion often arises in regard to such subjects as astrology or parapsychology. It is claimed that because we can collect statistics, run 'experiments' and construct 'theories' about such matters, the claims being made must be 'scientific' if not yet proven, and therefore ought to be taken seriously.

The truth, however, is that, in many cases at least, what is relevant to how we take such claims is not the method of investigating them but the nature of the questions to which the claims are purported answers. Thus the first question to ask about the like of the fork-bending Uri Geller is not 'Is it telekinesis?' but 'How does he do that trick?' And the appropriate person to answer that question is not a professional scientist but a professional magician; not Professor Taylor 'the respected scientist' but Ali Bongo 'the Great Magician'. Similarly, a scientist once claimed that it was irrational to believe in astrology because it had never been scientifically proven. As it were, it might be that the constellation of Scorpio influenced a twelfth of humanity but, as a matter of fact, it does not. In reality, the question being asked is much more like 'Could it be that men are influenced by square roots and women by fractions?'

When we are seeking to characterize the nature of science then, we must be aware that we are trying to distinguish it both from activities which are not scientific, and have no need to be, and from those which are scientific, and do need to be. Art history does not fail to do anything by not being science and nor does astrology achieve anything by pretending to be science. In short, science is interestingly different, in different ways, from both non-science and pseudo-science.

The traditional picture of science

If we piece together the traditional picture of science, what we arrive at is something like the following picture:

1 Realism
Science is an attempt to find out about one real world existing independently of all observers.

The truths it discovers about the world are truths, no matter what people happen to think about them.

There is only one best possible true description of any particular aspect of the world or of the world as a whole.

2 The distinction between observation and theory
Within science there is a fairly sharp distinction correctly drawn between reports of observations and statements of theory.

3 Observation reports are fundamental
Observations and experiments provide the foundations and justification for hypotheses and theories.

4 Precision of terms
Terms and concepts in both observation reports and statements of theory have clear, precise and unambiguous meanings.

5 Value-free
Terms and concepts in science have no normative (value-laden) content. Normative concepts have no place at all in science.

6 Testability
Scientific theories are tested by using experiments provisionally to determine the truths or certainly to determine the falsity of observation statements deduced from the theory.

7 Cumulative development
Science is cumulative in that, despite mistakes and blind alleys, science builds on what has been previously discovered.

8 Demarcation
There is a sharp distinction to be drawn between science and other ways of acquiring knowledge about the world. That there is such a distinction accounts for the enormous success of science over the last 400 years.

9 The unity of science

There should really be only one science about the one real world. Less profound sciences are reducible to more profound ones (psychology to biology, biology to chemistry, chemistry to physics). That science is now divided into different fields with differing methods is a consequence of our current ignorance.

The questions which arise about the bounds of science in this sense then are:

1 Are these claims tenable in their own right: *Could* science be like this?

2 Are these claims consistent with the history of science: *Is* science like this?

The different major philosophical theories of science from naive inductivism, through Popperian (Popper, 1963) falsificationism, to Kuhnian paradigm theories (Kuhn, 1970) to Lakatos' conception of the research programme (Latakos and Musgrove, 1970) take different views about these different questions.

Let us take one example. Is claim (2) tenable? That is, can it be part of scientific methodology that there is a sharp distinction between reports of observations and statements of theory? Two very different views of the nature of science give different answers to this question: the inductivist model and what we shall call the radical model of science.

THE INDUCTIVIST MODEL OF SCIENCE

One reason for thinking that there must be a sharp distinction between reports of observations and statements of theory is that this contrast forms a crucial part of the traditional image of science. According to it, the scientific observer with normal sense organs faithfully records what she hears, sees, etc. to be the case with respect to the experimental situation under observation and she does with a mind free of presuppositions. The observations are then recorded in 'observation statements' which are all singular statements, referring to some particular occurrence at a particular place and time. Thus such a statement might be:

At time *t* at place X, material of colour R was found and at time *t* + 1 at place X, another material of colour S was found.

On the traditional model, such singular statements are then generalized to form universal statements:

Whenever material of colour R is found, then material of colour S will also be found.

This process is called induction.

On one view, inductive reasoning is the key to scientific method. Perhaps something like this:

- All the facts are observed and recorded in a totally impartial manner.
- The observed facts are analysed and classified.

- From this analysis, generalizations are drawn about the relations between the facts.

This is the use of inductive reasoning. We have a limited number of facts, e.g. all As so far observed have been F and we then conclude that, probably, all As are F.

Since we can now have a law of the form 'All As are F' we can now use deductive reasoning to make a prediction, i.e. if all As are F is true, then the next observed A must be F. An experiment of further observation now confirms or disconfirms the truth of the prediction and hence of the deduction and hence of the original analysis and classification.

We can represent this picture of scientific method in Fig. 2. This picture of science is captured in the following passage:

> Everything that is science ultimately has its basis in the scientific method. Both the powers and the limitations of science are defined

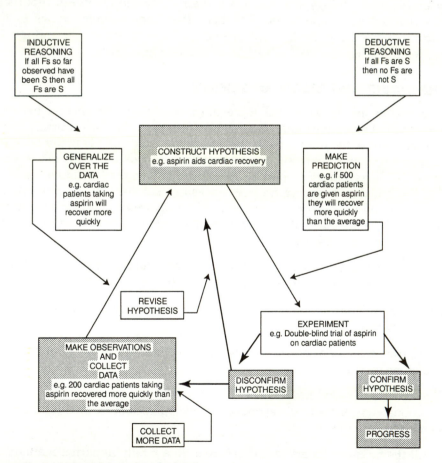

Figure 2 An inductivist model of science.

by this method. And wherever the scientific method cannot be applied, there cannot be science . . .

All science begins with observation, the first step of the scientific method. At once this delimits the scientific domain; something that cannot be observed cannot be investigated by science . . . It is necessary, furthermore, that an observation be repeatable, actually or potentially . . . Correct observation is a most difficult art, acquired only after long experience and many errors . . .

After an observation has been made, the second step of the scientific method is to define a problem. In other words, one asks a question about the observation. How does so and so come about? . . . More significantly, not everyone sees that there may actually be a problem connected with the observation . . . Anyone can ask questions. However, good questioning, like good observing, is a high art. To be valuable scientifically, a question must be relevant and it must be testable . . . Einstein's fame rests, in part, on showing that it is impossible to test whether or not the earth moves through an 'ether', an assumption held for many decades. All questions about an ether therefore become non-scientific, and we must reformulate associated problems until they become testable . . .

Having asked a proper question, the scientist proceeds to the third step of the scientific method. This involves the seemingly quite unscientific procedure of guessing. One guesses what the answer to the question might conceivably be. Scientists call this postulating a hypothesis . . . The scientist will not know whether his guess was or was not correct until he has completed the fourth step of the scientific method, experimentation. It is the function of every experiment to test the validity of a scientific guess . . . On the other hand, experiments do not guarantee a scientific conclusion. For there is ample room within experimentation and in succeeding steps to become unscientific again. Experimentation is by far the hardest part of scientific procedure. There are no rules to follow; each experiment is a case unto itself. Knowledge and experience usually help technically, but to design the experiment . . . that separates the genius from the dilettante . . . The result of any experiment represents evidence; that is the original guess in answer to a problem is confirmed as correct or is invalidated. If invalidated, a new hypothesis, with new experiments, must be thought up . . .

Experimental evidence is the basis for the fifth and final step in the scientific method, the formulation of a theory . . . Every good theory has predictive value. It prophesies certain results. In contrast to non-scientific prophecies, scientific ones always have a substantial body of evidence to back them up. Moreover, the scientific prophecy does not say that something will certainly happen but only that something is likely to happen, with a stated degree of probability.

With permission, Weisz, P.B., (1961)

This is the inductivist model of science. If enough singular statements occur then the general statement is testable by deducing consequences. Science works because it uses induction to generate testable hypotheses from certainly known observation statements and then uses deduction to test the truth of these hypotheses. This process clearly requires a sharp distinction between the reports of observations and statements of theory.

Can science work like this? Many philosophers have argued that it cannot. The sense perception upon which science is alleged to depend is not a matter of receiving information as if the scientist were a kind of magnetic tape, merely recording information in an entirely passive way. Rather, we know that we actively shape what we see in the light of the concepts we employ. This is true at the fundamental level of ordinary perception. For example, no one ever sees all sides of any object yet we take ourselves to be fully justified in saying that an object does have sides that we cannot see because that is precisely what the concept of an object involves.

At a more sophisticated level, we do not in any sense, envisaged by the claim under discussion, observe such things as 'chalk' in the world. This is shown if we are challenged in one's judgement that something is a piece of chalk. We will appeal to such statements as 'chalk leaves white marks when drawn against a blackboard'. Since other things might do this too, we might appeal to the fact that chalk, since it is composed of calcium carbonate, will produce carbon dioxide if immersed in acid. But how do we know that? Well, carbon dioxide turns lime water milky . . . At each challenge we have recourse to some further theoretical statement against the background of which we are justified in claiming that what we see before us now is a piece of chalk. Observations are theory-laden. But for this reason, observation statements cannot have the fundamental, foundational, role ascribed to them.

This is taken by some to undermine the objectivity of science and its claim to certainty. Others point out, in our view correctly, that it does no such thing – no more than the fact that we cannot see all sides of an object at once implies that we are not certain in our judgements that what we are now seeing is an object. Rather, it undermines only the claim that the objectivity of science is based on observation statements. Indeed, the view that the theory-ladenness of observation statements shares the assumption of its rival inductivist view. Both views hold that only rock-solid descriptions of what we observe can guarantee that our methods are objective.

But this assumption is mistaken. What we need is an account of the relation between observation statements and theories that stresses their mutual interdependence without forcing us into absurdity. The history of science gives us plenty of clues in this respect. Similar problems arise about every one of the traditional claims made about science. Indeed, against this traditional picture are ranged a set of theses which seek, either wholly or piecemeal, to undermine it.

The radical picture of science

1 Non-cumulativity
The history of science does not point to a linear gain in explanatory power but is characterized by discontinuities which result in explanatory loss and difference.

2 Theory-ladenness
Observation statements are not logically independent of theoretical statements.

3 Underdetermination
A given range of empirical observations is consistent with an indefinite number of theoretical explanations with the result that theories are always underdetermined by empirical data.

4 Holism
Statements can be tested against the empirical world only as parts of complete systems or nets of statements with the result that there is always available a choice about which statements to regard as disconfirmed.

5 Incommensurability
Empirical equivalent theories may not be inter translatable.

6 The non-epistemological character of emergence
There exist properties of complex systems which are not relations between those systems and something else, and cannot be derived from the properties attributable to the constituents of those systems whatever the degree of completeness of our knowledge of those constituents.

7 Social determinancy
Because science is a human, social activity, scientific beliefs are partly determined by social factors.

These objections to traditional views of science have been voiced by many. In particular, the final objection in our list, that science is determined by social factors, has gained wide currency. Those who call themselves 'social constructionists', for example, have developed a powerful argument to suggest that all science must be seen in terms of its cultural context. While this may be a useful critical stance to take, at its extreme it can be used as a justification for regarding scientific findings as no more than interesting cultural phenomena. For nursing, this position creates great difficulties as it seeks to develop a scientific basis for practice, particularly as science is seen as an antidote to traditional ineffective practices which owed more to the perpetuation of nursing rituals and culture than to proven worth. If science is just another cultural display, then are the results of science similarly suspect?

Great leaps forward

The second set of questions in the philosophy of science concerns 'bounds' in the sense of leaps. These questions amount to asking: 'What is the proper relation between the beliefs we acquire as the result of scientific inquiry and the beliefs that hold particularly central places in our everyday conceptual scheme?' Let us take two examples at the extremes to illustrate the problem.

We have the belief that the earth travels around the sun. We have no direct perceptual evidence for this, but we believe it about as firmly as we believe anything. If we are asked for evidence of this we will cite the history of physics, astronomy and cosmology. We believe this even though it still does seem to us that it is the sun that moves through the sky and we continue to use such phrases as 'sunrise' and 'sunset', even though we know that such terms are not literally in accord with the truth. In this case, we are aware that science directly contradicts our ordinary awareness and we are happy to accept that it is science and not our experience that is right.

But consider another example. The scientist Arthur Eddington wrote about two tables: one was the ordinary 'common-sense' table. This table was square with well-defined edges, brown in colour, having a smooth texture and, above all, was solid. The other table Eddington called his 'scientific table'. This table was colourless, textureless, merged gradually into the surrounding air and was composed almost entirely of empty space punctuated by atoms. Science has proved, wrote Eddington, that only the second table is real and that common sense is mistaken in believing that there are such things as solid tables in the world (Eddington, 1930).

What are we to say about this second suggestion that science directly conflicts with common sense? The shortest way with Eddington here is simply to agree with him. Henceforth, we say, we shall take science seriously and we shall refuse to use words such as 'solid' in regard to tables which bear no relation to how the world really is. Still Eddington will agree that, for convenience's sake, we still need a way of distinguishing parts of the world that will support typewriters, paper and cups of coffee and parts that will not. So, instead, we shall use the word 'zolid' where 'zolid' carries no implications about the actual physical composition of the objects it is applied to. We shall use such expressions as 'zolid as a rock' and 'Don't put your coffee there, it's not very zolid', and so on.

And now we ask: Has anything really changed? The answer is no. For our use of the world 'solid' did not, in itself, imply the truth or falsity of any scientific theory about what tables were actually composed of.

In short, Eddington cannot claim that physics has shown that the common-sense belief that tables are solid is false because at least one of the purposes of doing physics is to explain how there can be such things as solid tables at all by showing what they are made of. Here there is no real conflict between science and common sense.

The limitations of science

The third sense of 'bounds' delineating a set of questions in the philosophy of science is that of limitations. Are there questions which science cannot answer? We have seen that in a relatively trivial sense, there are such questions; that this is so is assumed in the very idea of scientific method in part being defined by a certain sort of question. Thus the question 'To what extent did the painter Marc Rothko escape from his surrealist origins?' is a perfectly respectable question admitting of an answer in art history but it is not a scientific question. No more than 'Shall I go to the cinema tonight?' is a question answerable by science.

But, equally, that science cannot answer such questions is no failure on its part; such questions do not impose limits on what science can achieve. Science simply does not ask such questions.

There are other questions which scientists can and do ask themselves but which, purely as scientists, cannot be answered by them. Typically ethical questions are of this form:

- 'Ought I to use animals in my research?'
- 'Ought I to accept military funding?'
- 'Ought I to juggle these experimental results so that I get the answer that I know is right?'

It is no good producing a research programme to answer these questions. What we need to recognize is that a scientist is not a special kind of person but a special kind of role. But again, this does not impose limits on the kinds of question that science can answer. The questions which are relevant here are those questions which, it is claimed, scientific inquiry can settle.

To take one example, it is often claimed today that we shall soon be able to build intelligent machines where, erroneously, it is thought that 'intelligence' also means 'self-consciousness' – the capacity to have mental states and awareness of mental states. The justification of this is the claim that the human mind stands to the human brain as computer programs stand to computer hardware – the mind is best understood as an information-processing system. Now the question of whether consciousness and the task that minds are able to carry out is best explained in terms of a computational model is not itself a scientific question. It is a conceptual question, one relevant to certain scientific enterprise but not one that can be settled simply by building machines on that hypothesis and seeing if they work. For deciding that they do 'work' in the relevant sense would beg the question at issue – what would we mean when we said that they 'worked'? In fact, the relation of mind to body is essentially a philosophical question with 2000 years of debate already behind it. It may well be that some of those engaged in research on artificial intelligence would do well to acquaint themselves with this debate before seeking funding on the basis of such extravagant and misleading claims. (There are many other examples of such questions where good science is thought to justify shabby philosophizing in a way that does science, philosophy and the lay public a grave disservice.)

So, while there are some questions which science would like to answer but cannot, we ought also to recognize that philosophy and science cannot be kept in separate isolation wards.

What kind of science does nursing need?

The above sections have provided some general sense of the sorts of questions which are the raw material of the philosophy of science, in terms of these three senses of the 'bounds of science': boundaries, leaps and limits. Clearly, only some of these questions are of any direct relevance to nursing science. But then it would be a poor scientist who was content to think of his or her work as completely isolated from other areas within science and therefore from the questions which arise about scientific activity as a whole. In an important sense, such an attitude would itself be profoundly unscientific. We now return to a more direct consideration of nursing, and the sort of science that it needs.

We have outlined the various positions which have been taken in the debate about the nature of science. These are fairly abstract points which seem to be more about the nature of science rather than its purpose. Talking about the purpose of science, however, raises a new set of problems which are connected to but slightly different from arguments about what it is. The purpose of science is variously described: there are some who see it as an end in itself – science as contemplation. Science does what it does for the sake of science, that is, increased knowledge about the world. Others take a less 'pure' view, and see the purpose of science (or, perhaps more correctly, the value of science) as being about the way in which scientific facts can be applied to problems in the world. This debate about 'pure' and 'applied' science has been rehearsed many times, and there is probably no need to go into it again. It is, however, difficult to think of what a pure science of nursing would look like, given that nursing is very much an applied discipline. Nurses do not, on the whole, spend all of their time in libraries or laboratories, but they do spend a lot of time nursing. This suggests that when we talk of a 'nursing science', we mean one which can be applied to nursing.

In order to think about ways of reconciling these views about science, therefore, it might be useful to think more carefully about the aims and practices of nursing, and then think about what sort of science it needs. Thinking about forms of science, and then trying to fit nursing into them, seems to be putting the cart before the horse.

At this point, it might be useful to make a distinction between 'knowing about nursing' and 'nursing knowledge'. For the purposes of this debate, 'nursing knowledge' is defined as the knowledge, information, or understanding that nurses need to do the job. Examples would be knowledge about wound healing, pain control or counselling strategies. 'Knowledge about nursing' is knowledge about the job itself – the way nurses manage their tasks, the way they are constrained or enabled by various factors, their aims and aspirations. Both types of knowledge are important, and are, of course interrelated. Moreover, the same debates apply to the best way to acquire these types of knowledge, in other words what a science of nursing should look like. Before we go on to examine the characteristics of nursing practice (and therefore the type of knowledge required), then, we will briefly discuss the problems of finding out what they are. This illustrates the way in which knowledge about nursing and nursing knowledge are related, and also the general debates which are held about the nature of science.

Knowledge about nursing

Characteristics of nursing have been identified from a number of sources. Firstly, there is the experience of nurses, as revealed in conversations and discussions with them. Secondly, there is the empirical evidence available from research studies which have examined nursing activity from a variety of methodological perspectives. Thirdly, there is the prescriptive writing of nurses (and others) which has sought to present what nursing should be, or in other words what good nursing would look like. The 'goodness' of this nursing is variously described as being 'effective', 'professional' or 'caring', and each of these terms is open to further examination, but nonetheless these notions of good nursing have gained a wide currency in nursing theory and policy. It is likely, therefore, that they have had some impact on actual practice.

These three sources of information about nursing have different values according to the view of the people receiving such information, and this in itself is an interesting point to explore. Conversations with nurses could be called 'anecdotal' evidence and dismissed by those who value more systematic, objective or representative enquiry, while it is valued by those who regard experientially gained knowledge 'straight from the horse's mouth' as being a more direct form of understanding. Research data are similarly subject to varying esteem, partly in relation to anecdotal evidence, but also according to which methodological approach has been employed in the study. Research findings, therefore, can either be decried as decontextualized and abstract if it is reductionist and the reader is not, or it can be regarded as woolly and imprecise if it is qualitative and the reader is not. Prescriptions for nursing, no matter how logically derived, can be decried by both the research and the anti-research lobby on the basis of the values that they imply. It can be argued that these values are not shared by everyone, or that this writing demonstrates a confusion between facts and values. Again, these caveats arise partly from the tensions between the positions taken about the respective merits of subjective and objective knowledge about nursing. The 'subjectivists' can challenge nursing ideals on the basis that they ignore variations in the ideals of individual nurses and patients, and the 'objectivists' object to nursing ideals because they have no factual, objective basis and disguise polemic as science.

That many of these nursing ideals are called 'nursing theory', only adds to the confusion – what sort of theory are they? In the discussion above, we outlined different views of theory, and we can apply these now. If nursing theories are theories in the traditional view of science, then they should be value-free, precise, based on systematic observation, testable and universally applicable. It is arguable that few, if any, nursing theories meet these criteria. If they are not traditional theories, then they fare a little better, but they fail to acknowledge their socially situated nature, and therefore to make their construction clear.

This discussion on the relative worth of different ways of knowing about nursing is directly related to the questions posed in this chapter, as it demonstrates the debates which rage over the purpose and nature of science. Leaving this debate aside for the moment, however, we will go on to look at nursing practice as it is described anecdotally, by research, and by prescriptive theory, in order to examine the implications of this practice for the development of nursing knowledge and science.

Characteristics of nursing

HOLISTIC PRACTICE

Nursing theories have generally described nursing as involving physiological, psychological and social aspects of health and health care. In other words, they propose that nursing care should not focus solely on the physical aspects of health and disease, but take account of the psychological and social consequences and contexts of health problems. Nursing an elderly person with diabetes, for example, does not simply present a physiological problem, which can be addressed by adjustment of diet and medication, but also involves assessment and intervention in other areas. Care may therefore involve education, in that the person may need to learn more about their problem; counselling, in that the person may feel stigmatized or anxious; and practical help and advice, in that the social and financial circumstances of the person may make adherence to a treatment regime difficult.

The fundamental principle behind holistic nursing care is that all of these aspects of health are interrelated, and cannot be separated. It is therefore important, if nursing care is to be successful in helping people to gain or maintain health, that nursing care develops strategies to address these aspects. This makes sense on 'common-sense' or experiential grounds – stories abound of patients whose anxiety about their illness creates more problems than the illness itself, or patients who did not understand their medication or medical advice, or patients whose social circumstances either led to their health problems or prevented recovery. There is also research evidence which has linked social circumstances with health problems (occupational hazards, poor diet and stress, for example, have been linked with particular lifestyles), and psychological phenomena with somatic problems (for example, the increased need for analgesia in post-operative patients who are anxious).

If we accept the notion of holistic nursing as being a logical way to practice, however, we are then faced with the problem of developing nursing knowledge from a wide range of scientific traditions. If we link aspects of holistic nursing to the academic disciplines which underpin them, we find that each discipline has a very different view of the proper way to develop science. The physical aspects of care are informed by research and theory which takes place in the arena of the physical sciences: physiology, microbiology, pharmacology, medical physics and radiology to name but a few of the many branches of the life sciences. These correspond most closely to the traditional view of science outlined earlier, in that they are all concerned with value-free empirical study which is testable and objective. Looking at other aspects of care, however, we find that the criteria for good science are not unanimous. Within the disciplines of psychology and, perhaps more so, sociology, there are major differences in the way that science is practised and regarded. The debate is usually characterized as being between the quantitative and qualitative researchers (the names vary from dispute to dispute but these are the terms most frequently applied).

At the risk of stereotyping these positions, the positions can be summarized thus: quantitative researchers argue that the criteria which are used in the physical sciences should apply to research done in the area of human phenomena, whereas qualitative researchers argue that there is a difference between the two areas of study which should be reflected in the methodology used. Qualitative researchers come closest to the anti-traditionalist position outlined above.

These myriad methodological positions can lead to nurses using research findings which arise from incompatible and antagonistic views of science. When helping a patient with pain, for example, a nurse can draw upon physiological and pharmaceutical science to understand pain mechanisms and the effect of analgesia, and also, perhaps, qualitative sociological research which has described how patients can either have their pain legitimized or dismissed by nurses because of the expectations that they have of different illness trajectories. Nurses can, and do, synthesize different types of science in their everyday work, and do not worry too much about the debates that might occur if the researchers whose work they draw upon were to be invited to debate the relative merits of their methodology. However, this eclectic use of science glosses over the differences in scope, aims and intentions of the various bodies of work that they refer to.

DECISION-MAKING IN NURSING

Another aspect of nursing, which is perhaps the one which is of greatest importance to practitioners, is the need for nurses to make decisions about care. These may be life or death decisions, such as the decision about the best way to stop a haemorrhage, or they may be less urgent, such as the point at which a catheter needs changing or the need to give analgesia. Nevertheless, the decisions that nurses make have important consequences for patients, and in making them the nurse may well feel the need for some certainty or clear recommendations from research.

Decision-making is not just simply a matter of nurses needing some sort of reassurance that the actions that they take will be safe and helpful, although this may well be a part of their concern. It is also a matter of knowing that actions do have effects, and that some are therapeutic and some are injurious. In other words, while some research will highlight the relativity or context-bound nature of some aspects of human life, like individual manifestations of pain or embarrassment, there are other aspects which are difficult to see as relative. Such absolute aspects tend to be physiological phenomena – death, for example, is not relative – but others, such as fear, anger, hostility, though they may have some element of social construction, undoubtedly do happen.

Seeing all science as simply a cultural phenomenon and subject to varying interpretations may well be, at times, a useful critical stance to take. It does not, however, always help nurses to decide on action to take when faced with the suffering of patients. In these situations, then, it is tempting to believe that there is, indeed, a value-free science which can tell us what is 'really real'.

NURSING CARE AS INDIVIDUALIZED CARE

Alongside holism in nursing runs a complementary theme, which is the idea that nursing care should not only respect the entirety of the experiences of patients, but that it should do so on an individual basis. In other words, principles of holism cannot be applied wholesale to patients as a class of people, but only as unique individuals. Respecting the individual circumstances and preferences of patients, however, depends on finding out what these are, and incorporating them into any plans for care. Not only is this knowledge sometimes difficult to obtain and act upon, but it also raises the possibility of conflicts between patients and nurses, particularly when ideologies conflict. If nurses become firmly wedded to the view that their knowledge is scientific and therefore, as we discussed earlier, 'better', then the non-scientific beliefs of patients become little more than subjects of scientific study rather than incorporated into care. In other words, nurses will study lay beliefs in order to see how their effect on care can be moderated or overcome – they will be seen as barriers to scientific care rather than contributions.

One body of work which has sought to treat the views of patients as more than conceptual oddities has been the anti-psychiatry movement, which flew a brave flag for the patients voice. Writers and practitioners such as R.D. Laing, for example, argued that the things that people who had been called 'schizophrenic' said were perfectly valid ways of viewing the world, rather than pathologies to be treated. The arguments of the anti-psychiatry movement seem to have been crushed under the weight of the psycho-biologists, but there are traces of this position to be found in the consumerism evident in health-care debates today. Consumerism as a manifestation of capitalist society is unlikely to have direct links with the radical anti-psychiatry movement of the 1960s and 1970s, but they do, surprisingly, both support the voice of the client, often in preference to that of the professional.

Discussion and conclusion

Nursing practice, then, presents several challenges for the development of a nursing science. The need for 'facts' which will guide decision-making suggests that at one level nurses need to support the traditional view of science as objective and value-free – there is no room to entertain suspicions about research findings as being anything else. The demands of holistic care, however, suggest that nursing science needs to embrace a number of academic disciplines, some of which will not conform to the traditional view of science, and indeed will form its strongest critics. Individualized care puts this problem into even sharper focus with the potential for direct conflict between scientific and non-scientific beliefs about health care.

One of the ways out of this dilemma, which has been suggested by some (see, for example Virginia Henderson's discussion of the nursing process; Henderson, 1982) is to see nursing practice as being both scientific and artistic. This view of the artistry of nursing regards some of the things that nurses do as 'craft' and therefore, presumably, subject to aesthetic debate rather than scientific discussion. This view seems to owe a great deal to traditional notions of science – the areas of nursing which are described as artistry are usually activities such as developing relationships with patients and managing care; the first has been more usually addressed by non-traditional science, and the second belongs to applied rather than pure forms. The idea of dividing nursing into the domains of art and science, then, does not really address the nature of nursing science; it simply defines the limits of science in a particular way.

Another option is to reject the notion of nursing science altogether, and view all practice as craft. Again, however, this rests on the traditional notion of science as objective and abstract. The anti-science argument rests partly on the grounds that such an abstract science is incongruent with the very practical and often emotional nature of nursing, which indeed it is. Another anti-science argument is related to the commendatory aspect of the term 'scientific' which we discussed earlier in this chapter. The claims of nursing to be scientific are therefore regarded with suspicion as being claims to a higher status for nursing. It is somewhat disturbing that nurses should castigate themselves for claiming more respect for what they do, but the argument is a little more understandable if it is reduced to its constituent stages, which seem to be:

- Nurses should nurse for the sake of their patients not for personal glory. Therefore,
- if nurses seek personal glory, they are nursing for themselves and not for patients.

The search for scientific status, therefore, becomes an aspiration which forgets the 'real' business of nursing.

There are a number of problems with this argument, not least the difficulty in accepting that the desires of nurses and patients have to be antagonistic, that one group will only ever gain at the expense of the other. There are, however, some grounds for agreeing that if nurses want nursing science only for the status it brings them, then it is not likely that this science will be developed in order to meet patients' needs (although it may do accidentally). This may be particularly the case if the science being sought is traditional science, which exists for itself and its practitioners, rather than the applied, culturally embedded science which has, until fairly recently, enjoyed less academic status.

The anti-science arguments in nursing seem to be based on the traditional notion of science as abstract, objective and pure. As such, these arguments do have some weight, but if the notion of science is changed, then the arguments become weaker. If nursing science broadens its definition to incorporate critiques of traditional science, then it becomes possible to think about a science which is part of the social world, rather than separate from it, which can accommodate different explanations of events, and acknowledges the values which underpin it. This sort of science seems to fit nursing better than the traditional description.

But can we do this? Can we simply select the bits of science that we like, and add on bits that we think are missing without creating something very different? Would the thing that we create bear little resemblance to the thing that we started with, and therefore become a nonsense? What other problems would arise from this 'new science'? This problem is related to the different positions which we outlined earlier, which can be described in this way:

Traditionalists
Science is X (where X = objective, value-free, etc.)

Critics
Not only is science not X, but X is not possible.

While it may be possible to live with the idea that science is not X, the idea that X is not possible creates more serious problems. By treating all science as simply a social occupation and therefore a particular view of the world with no greater claim to truth than any other, we find ourselves in a world where everything is uncertain, indeed where certainty cannot exist. For nurses faced with decisions to make, and things to do, the idea that the basis of their actions is just another story about the world is very disconcerting. What is needed is a middle way between the opposing views of science. The anti-traditional view of science can be a useful cautionary check to passive acceptance of scientific findings, while the traditional view of science can be seen as a description (though flawed) of the process by which particular results were produced. Evaluating findings, therefore, becomes a matter of placing scientific work in the context of the general qualifications which can be made about science *per se*, and the particular conditions which science aims to meet. When faced with a particular question, therefore, nurses need to ask whether it is a question for science, and if so, whether science has answered it in the way that science does. If nurses decide that this is the case, then the answers that science has provided need to be seen in the context of the culture in which it has provided them.

This middle way seems a little weak, hedged with qualifications and caveats; in short, it does not tell us what can be regarded as true and what as false. Perhaps, however, faith that there can be absolute certainty (never mind that science can provide it) is somewhat misguided. This is, perhaps, a metaphysical question, but it may be useful here to remember the words of Keats who, in a letter to his brother used the term 'negative capability' which he defined as being 'the faculty of not having to make up one's mind about everything'. Negative capability may seem, at first, to be an evasion of responsibility for nurses – one can imagine nurses with negative capability responding to calls for help and advice with philosophical shrugs of their shoulders. Negative capability, however, is a useful notion, in that it suggests that decisiveness is not an unqualified virtue, and that there may be more merit in regarding knowledge (and science) as indicative rather than definitive.

References

Eddington, A.S. 1930: *The nature of the physical world*. Cambridge: Cambridge University Press.
Henderson, V. 1982: The nursing process – is the title right? *Journal of Advanced Nursing 7*, 103–9.
Kuhn, T.S. 1970: *The structure of scientific revolutions*. Chicago: University of Chicago Press.
Lakatos, I. and Musgrove, A. 1970: *Criticism and the growth of knowledge*. Cambridge: Cambridge University Press.
Popper, K. 1963: *Conjectures and refutations*. London: Routledge and Kegan Paul.
Weisz, P.B. 1961: *Elements of biology*. New York: McGraw–Hill.

Further reading

Ayer, A.J. 1972: *Probability and evidence*. London: Macmillan.
Blackburn, S. 1973: *Reason and prediction*. Cambridge: Cambridge University Press.
Butler, S. 1981: *Life and habit*. London: Wildwood House.
Calder, N. 1982: *Einstein's Universe: the layman's guide*. Harmondsworth: Pelican.
Capra, F. 1976: *The Tao of physics*. Glasgow: Fontana.
Chalmers, A.F. 1976: *What is this thing called science?* Milton Keynes: Open University Press.
Chant, C. and Fauvel, J. 1980: *Historical studies on science and belief*. Milton Keynes: Open University Press.

Coveney, P. and Highfield, R. 1991: *The arrow of time.* London: Flamingo.
Darwin, C. 1911: *The origin of species.* London: Watts.
Feynman, R. 1983: *The character of physical law.* Cambridge, MA: MIT Press.
Hacking, I. 1981: *Scientific revolutions.* Oxford: Oxford University Press.
Huff, D. 1954: *How to lie with statistics.* Harmondsworth: Pelican.
Kant, I. 1928: *The critique of judgement.* Oxford: Oxford University Press.
Laudan, L. 1990: *Science and relativism – some key controversies in the philosophy of science.* Chicago: University of Chicago Press.
Magee, B. 1973: *Popper.* Glasgow: Fontana.
Midgley, M. 1989: *Wisdom, information and wonder – what is knowledge for?* London: Routledge and Kegan Paul.
Midgley, M. 1992: *Science as salvation – a modern myth and its meaning.* London: Routledge and Kegan Paul.
Rescher, N. 1978: *Scientific progress.* Oxford: Basil Blackwell.
Rose, H. and Rose, S. 1970: *Science and society.* Harmondsworth: Pelican.
Warnock, M. 1984: *Report of the Committee of Inquiry into Human Fertilisation and Embryology.* London: HMSO.
Waterfield, R. 1989: *Before eureka.* Bristol: Bristol Classical Press.
Weisz, P.B. 1969: *Elements of biology,* 3rd edn. New York: McGraw–Hill.

Philosophy of mind

5

INTRODUCTION

One of the central tenets of nursing theory, of whatever kind, is the assertion that nurses need to treat the patient as an individual, with unique characteristics, needs, strengths and problems. This is justified on pragmatic grounds, as the best way to ensure appropriate and efficient care, but also on ethical and philosophical grounds as the way to ensure that care incorporates respect for the person. Similarly and additionally, nurses have expressed support for ideas of partnership in care, where care is negotiated with the patient, rather than imposed on them, and where patient education and information enables this to happen.

Throughout these discussions, the nature of the patient is almost taken for granted. The patient is a competent person, able to make decisions once information is provided, and if for reasons of temporary incapacity the patient is unable to do so, then nurses can make predictions of what they would decide if they were able. This view of persons, however, runs some risks of assuming too much about the preferences of patients and, perhaps more importantly, fails to tackle the issue of what it means to be a person. Many patients do not fit the rational, reasonable model of personhood (and neither do many nurses!), not just because they are ill, but because rationality is not all there is to being a person. The danger is, therefore, that if we use normative models of personhood, with their emphasis on reason and rationality, we may exclude some people from this definition, and because of their lack of reason deny their personhood.

This paves the way for abuses of patients, excused on the grounds that professionals know best about what is good for them, but even when action is benevolent and well intentioned, there are many debates which should arise for nurses. Firstly, there is the question of what it means to be a person, and secondly there is the question of how persons should be treated. In holistic nursing, where a person is seen as a complex whole with mental and physical characteristics, we have problems when one of these sets of characteristics is missing or impaired, and it is interesting to note that it is problems of mental function which call personhood most into question. If we imagine such a thing as a disembodied mind, something which, as far as we know has never occurred outside the world of science fiction, it may seem relatively easy to still think of this mind as being a person. If, however, we think of a mindless body, it is much more difficult to think of it as being an individual. Despite the evident physical phenomenology of living, physicality is not enough to define personhood. The mindless bodies that we do encounter outside nursing, the primitive insects and algae, and, of course, in the vegetable kingdom, are not usually credited with personhood, and when confronted with a mindless body in nursing (or even a body with an impaired mind) the temptation is to treat them in the same way, as vegetables.

Take, for example, the case of a person with Alzheimer's disease, cared for in a nursing home. This person may be relatively physically fit, able to walk around, and care for themselves to a considerable degree. If this person, however, 'wanders' from the care facility, this will cause some consternation in the staff, and efforts will be made to prevent this. If the person repeatedly asserts that they want to leave, and argues that the staff have no right to stop them, then this will not be taken seriously enough to allow the person to go. If this person, five minutes after an escape attempt, sits down quietly to watch television, and seems to have forgotten the incident, this will be taken as evidence that he or she did not 'really' mean it.

A person with Alzheimer's disease has two kinds of cognitive problem. There is a reduced ability to function intellectually, to reason, to cope with information, and to make decisions. Underlying this, however, is a second problem, to do with short-term memory; indeed, this is often the problem that clinches a diagnosis of Alzheimer's disease. Short-term memory loss means that information cannot be processed and retained; people with Alzheimer's disease will forget that they have just had meals, or that a friend has been to visit, or that they have just been angry. A few minutes later, they may ask when lunch will be, or why no-one has been to see them, or be cheerful and pleasant.

This lack of short-term memory makes a person with Alzheimer's disease very difficult to regard as a person, if part of personhood involves some form of stability. Without memory, which links the past to the present, there is no continuity of action, knowledge, attitude, or, we may think, feeling. The person with Alzheimer's disease can therefore seem little more than a roulette wheel of random responses to the world, and this does not fit with ideas of personhood which involve consistency. For something to be identified as a person, we expect it to remain recognizable as that person over time.

These questions about personhood lie at the heart of nursing, its ethical foundations and its clinical practice. The ethical debates about personhood involve definitions of the moral nature of such a state, and furthermore, debates about how persons should act towards each other. In philosophical thought there is therefore a substantial body of work which has addressed these issues, and, not surprisingly arrived at different ideas of personhood according to the ethical systems in which the debate is located. In other words, different concepts of what it is to be a person may underlie different moral viewpoints. For example, faced with thinking about determining public policy in health care, the moral viewpoint we may have to adopt is one that puts the individuality of the beneficiaries or victims of that policy to one side (Ground and Hughes, 1996). Thus, insofar as utilitarian thinking enters in here, 'person' is thought of as the name of a collection of experiences of states – some good, some bad – which are thought of as essentially transferable. Roughly speaking, more happiness in one collection can compensate for more misery in another. As it were, it is what is in the container, not the container itself, which is important.

Faced with thinking about particular individuals and their needs however, we cannot use the same picture. Here the 'container' is primary. So much so that, for some people, the continued existence of the container is desirable no matter what the quality of its contents. Here it seems that nothing done or not done to one individual can compensate for anything done or not done to someone else.

Neither of these ways of thinking is wrong, but they do clash and we need to understand when and why they do. Different conceptions of what it is to be a person result in disagreements about what we ought to do in particular cases. Furthermore, even agreed conceptions of what it is to be a person can fall apart when we are faced with particular sorts of illness. Probably the most widespread examples of this problem occur in the treatment of people who have learning difficulties or a mental illness. We need to face up to the problems of why it is that we can find it so difficult to include these human beings within the parameters of our ordinary capacities for respect of persons. The problem arises because we think it important to accord all human beings the respect we normally accord to persons. But in many cases we find it difficult to see how the concept of personhood can apply. The fear is that to withdraw the application of the concept of person would be to render our respect for them and therefore the resources we allocate to them unjustifiable. It may be, however, that we would do better to reconsider how we treat objects of moral concern which are not persons. As we will discuss at the end of this chapter, using the notion of 'human beings' rather than 'persons' allows a less restricted application of the principle of respect.

The philosophy of mind has two main concerns. Firstly, there is the relationship between mind and body; in other words, whether the mind is simply a physiological phenomenon, made up of chemical reactions in the brain, or whether mental life is of a quite different order. The second, and related, concern is about the place of the mind in definitions of personhood; in other words, whether persons can be defined in terms of their mental life alone, or whether some cognisance must be taken of their physical life.

It is the second of these concerns that will form the basis of the discussion in this chapter which illustrates the range of theories about personhood and looks at their central arguments and problems. We start with a general consideration of how the adequacies of these theories can be assessed and what criteria they must meet to be considered 'adequate'. To illustrate these theories, we have included a number of 'thought experiments' which are essentially hypothetical situations in which personhood is explored.

Theories of philosophy of mind

There are essentially two sorts of theory which seek to explain what it is to be a person. This not to say that such kinds of theories are mutually exclusive or that a single theory may not contain elements of both, only that it is useful to distinguish them in the following way (the two theories are further expanded upon below).

Normative theories

These theories state what are alleged to be necessary condition of person-hood by using concepts which are value-based. These can be either ethical concepts or else concepts which rely upon accepted notions of correctness and incorrectness. For example, the capacity for being rational often figures in such accounts but what counts as being 'rational' depends upon accepted standards or norms of correctness, validity, etc. Because of their use of *normative* concepts, this sort of theory is commonly supposed to be of particular relevance to the moral problems which involve making decisions about the concept of person we should employ. In practice, however, such theories only rarely avoid either begging the question at stake in such issues or relying on imported non-normative elements.

Non-normative theories

These theories state what are alleged to be necessary and sufficient conditions of personhood. In large part they all depend on the following methodological idea:

> The conditions of a thing's identity over time depend upon what sort of thing it is.

> Therefore to know the conditions of a thing's identity over time is to know what sort of thing it is.

So, if we knew what changes someone could undergo and still remain the same person, we could find out what changes someone could not undergo and still remain the same person.

Because these theories are interested in establishing necessary conditions of being a person, they distinguish between the factors which we simply happen to use to identify someone as the 'same person' from those factors which we must use.

It is easy to see this distinction if we think of a totalitarian society where people are always identified by the identity card they carry. It would not follow that being a person consisted in having an identity card. This is just what complaints about being deemed a 'non-person' by such regimes are based upon – there is more to being a person than being a citizen.

In order to isolate these necessary features of personhood, these theories often have recourse to imaginary and often bizarre thought experiments called 'survival test-cases' (we include some examples at the end of this chapter). They are usually of the form 'Would you survive as a person if . . .'. If you think that you would not survive the ordeal described, then you would seem to believe that the situation described involves a change in some necessary condition of being the same person.

The status of these stories is itself problematic. Some philosophers believe that these stories prove nothing. But it is hard to say just why this should be. In addition, it may be that rejecting these survival test cases has more disturbing implications for our concept of person than accepting them.

Despite these disagreements, however, the general idea that understanding 'same person' will enable us to understand 'person' is widely accepted. Both sorts of theory must meet at least the following conditions:

1 The theory must account for at least the central features of both the first- and the third-person perspective. In other words, it must fit in with how we think about our own personhood and that of others.

2 The theory must be non-circular in that it does not assume the truth of its own conclusion. (A general requirement of any theory, of course, but one which is particularly hard to meet in the case of talk about 'person'.)

3 The theory must allow, at least in principle, for the possibility of non-human persons, in a way that avoids the circularity of saying simply that 'humans are persons'.

4 If the theory is in conflict with any of our intuitions concerning the nature of persons, then it must explain why the relevant intuition is independently demonstrable as incoherent and/or appeal to intuition in general is irrelevant or unjustifiable.

5 Any normative concepts employed in the theory must be fundamental, i.e. not reducible to other concepts whose application are themselves problematic.

6 The theory must be able to deal with an adequate range of survival test cases or else explain why such cases are individually or generally irrelevant.

7 The theory must not employ arguments which would make the identity of material objects over time problematic.

8 The theory must be at least consistent with accepted empirical data or explain why such data have been incorrectly described or interpreted.

9 The theory cannot be wholly normative if it is inconsistent with some possible non-normative theory and vice versa.

Normative theories

Unlike non-normative theories, normative theories of personhood are not easily classifiable. What we find instead are variations on a loose group of themes. These themes include:

- Language use
- Acting according to laws or rules
- Moral relations with others
- Attitudes towards life as a whole
- Autonomy
- Holding rights
- Being able to make claims against others
- Self-determination
- Objects of respect for their own sake
- Self-reflective judgements

Two classical exponents of this approach are Locke and Kant. Locke distinguished 'person' from 'man', arguing that the latter was what we would now call a biological term whilst the former was a 'forensic' term, that is, a term related to issues that could arise in a court of law: responsibility, culpability, and so on. Having established that 'person' was thus a normative concept, he went on to argue that the term applies only to 'intelligible agents capable of a law, and happiness and misery' (*An essay concerning human understanding*, Book II, chapter 27).

The notion of law also plays an important part in the account of 'person' offered by Immanuel Kant. For Kant, a person is something capable of self-legislation, i.e. capable of creating rules for itself which, having been created, are understood as necessary constraints on action. (Note that Kant also had much to say about non-normative theories of personhood.)

The principal insights of this sort of theory can be summarized as follows:

- The guiding idea that the concept of 'person' is an amalgam of factual and moral notions is a compelling one. It is certainly right to point out that we cannot decide the question of whether or not something is a person simply by staring at it long enough.
- This sort of theory would appear to have a particular relevance to the moral problems which involve the concept of 'person'.
- For the most part, this sort of theory does not have recourse to the bizarre thought experiments that occur in non-normative theories.

In general, this sort of theory fails to meet conditions (1), (4), (5) and (8). Particular theories often fail to meet conditions (2) and (5). The failures can be summarized as follows:

- From the fact that we cannot tell simply through straightforward empirical investigation whether or not something is a person, it does not follow that the non-factual elements in the concept of person must be moral ones. This is so even if judging that something is a person commits us to certain sorts of moral relation to it.
- Too often, the theory's normative concepts depend upon unarticulated non-normative assumptions. This is most evident when the theory begins to talk about capacities or potential for rationality, moral relations with others, etc. Should the person or thing that has the potential not be more important than just the potential itself?

- Equally problematic is the fact that, at least very often, such theories are of no help in deciding particular moral questions about people. This is because the theories are often constructed just in order to arrive at a particular solution to a moral issue. But to the claim 'Embryos count as persons' it seems all too easy to reply, 'If so, why is research on embryos permissible?'. One seems left with the clash between intuitions which caused the problem in the first place.

One way of dividing up normative theories of person is to look at the arguments made about where personhood resides, in other words what is taken to be the central location of the person, which is independent of any vagaries of other parts of life. We have divided theories, therefore, into theories which focus on the soul (a non-physical transcendent aspect of the human condition), experience (the activities and events of a person's life) and the body (the physical structure of a person). Each of these theories has different consequences for the way in which a person can be defined.

Soul

These theories can be summarized as the claim that a person is a substance which has the following properties:

- It is not physical and is therefore distinct from the body.
- It is not spatially located though it does have temporal location.
- It is simple and therefore indivisible. Hence its survival is all or nothing and not a matter of degree.
- Its survival consists in nothing other than its identity over time.
- It is not reducible to any other entity or any set of relations. In particular, it is not reducible to the mental states of which it is the subject.
- It is the object to which 'I' refers.
- Its nature is revealed only from the first person perspective.
- It affects and can be affected by physical states of the body. Therefore physical change can be evidence for, though it cannot constitute, its existence and non-existence.

Many exponents of this type of theory belong to the tradition of dualism which argues for the separation of the mind and the body. This move, however, tends to portray the person as having two separate sorts of life, which is contrary to our intuitions. Dualism proper is Cartesian dualism as propounded by Descartes, discussed in Chapter 3. But Leibniz and Malebranche were also famous exponents of other variants of dualism. One enthusiastic if surprising modern exponent is Sir John Eccles, the Nobel Prize winning neurophysiologist, in *The Self and its Brain*.

The principal insights of the theory can be summarized as follows:

- The theory seems to do full justice to our intuitions about ourselves as seen from the first-person perspective.
- It is consistent with, and supportive of, many of our ethical and religious beliefs.
- It provides an explanation of the difference between mental and physical concepts.

The failures of the theory, however, are as follows (see conditions (1), (5) and (7):

- Third-person knowledge of persons becomes a matter of inference. The theory, therefore, does not meet the first condition set out previously, in that it does not account for the third-person perspective in that we might be able to know our own personhood, but not that of others.
- The problem of how the soul can affect and be affected by the body appears insuperable. The theory does not therefore meet condition (5), in that it infers some sort of connection between the soul and the body, which is problematic.
- The connection between the existence of an object – any object, even an immaterial object – and my own survival, is problematic in the extreme. This does not meet condition (7) in that it fails to adequately describe survival of the person over time.

Experience

A person is a set of mental states related in certain appropriate ways such that:

- The existence of the appropriate relations between mental states at different times constitutes the identity of a person over time.
- The appropriate relations are causal with memory playing the crucial role.
- The existence of such relations is not all or nothing but a matter of degree. Hence the question of whether or not a person survives some changes may not admit of a determinate answer.
- There is no essence of a person which is available either from a first-person or a third-person point of view. Since there is nothing to have a special perspective of this kind on its own states, there is nothing available from the first-person point of view that is not also available from the third-person point of view. There are only more or less complicated mental states. Consequently 'I' does not refer to any object but is simply the expression of a mental state which refers to its relations with other mental states.
- Since a person is constituted by the content of mental states and the relations between them, the fact that these relations are causal and, therefore have a particular physical basis, is irrelevant. The mental states could have the same content and the same relations to each other even if the physical basis were a different object and worked in different ways.

- The concept of a person does not obey the common-sense rules of identity governing ordinary objects. But this can be explained. Persons are like clubs or nations. What is important is not identity, but survival. Unlike identity, survival may be partial and, over the whole course of a person's life, is partial.

The so called 'bundle theory', that persons are a bundle of experiences, properly belongs to Hume (see *A treatise of human nature*, part IV, section VI). Derek Parfit is the modern evangelist for this theory, holding that virtually the whole of ethics is based on a bias towards egoism and the pursuit of self-interest because of our failure to accept this view of ourselves. Ethics cannot be put on a rational basis until the ego is taken out of egoism (see Parfit's *Reasons and persons*).

The principal insights of the theory are as follows:

- The theory very successfully exposes the illusion that the nature of what it is to be a person could be revealed through a special kind of inward looking at oneself. This does indeed have radical consequences for our understanding of 'person'.
- It is consistent with empirical data in that it can account for the strange dislocation of our ordinary concept of person in the case of persons suffering from brain damage and other dysfunctions. (In *The man who mistook his wife for a hat*, the neurologist Oliver Sacks refers to people suffering from Korsakov's syndrome as 'Humean beings'.) The difference between these tragic cases and ourselves is here a matter of degree, not of kind.
- Though radically at odds with many Western ethical and religious beliefs, for some people, the theory appears to have a compelling consolatory aspect akin to some Eastern religions. Using this theory, it is possible to give a sense to the claim that we need not be so concerned as we are about our own inevitable deaths and that there are no absolute barriers between self and others. (Others, of course, find both these ideas quite horrifying.)

It is difficult to identify inadequacies of the theory because its failure to meet some of the conditions of any adequate theory is thought by its exponents to be amongst its principal virtues. They take the imposition of such conditions to be errors based on illusions for which they offer explanations as part of the theory being advanced. Dissatisfaction with the theory is best put forward at this level:

- The theory does not sufficiently explain why our intuitions about our own nature should be so radically and systematically mistaken (condition (1)).
- It is not clear that we can really give any sense to the idea of mental states which do not have a subject in the sense traditionally understood. This is in conflict with our intuitions, but the theory does not really explain why this intuition is mistaken (condition (4)).
- The theory finds it difficult to account for survival test cases involving amnesia or radical personality changes. It is difficult, however, to press this point because of the danger of begging the question concerning the correctness of our intuitions (condition (6)).

Body

This theory has two major forms:

A person is a living body.
A person is a particular part of a living body, namely the brain.

Therefore:

- The identity of a person consists in the physical or biological continuity of the body (brain).
- The body (brain) meets some independently derivable minimum conditions of proper function.
- Though, in principle, such continuity is a matter of degree, in practice the survival or a body (brain) is all or nothing.
- But since the question of whether or not some body (brain) meets the conditions of proper function may not admit of a definite answer, the question of whether or not someone is the same person may not admit of a definite answer. Hence it is possible that whether or not something is a person at all may not admit of a definite answer.
- The identity of a person over time is independent of the continuity of the mental states which the body (brain) causally subserves. Hence the fact that someone may sincerely claim that they are some particular person does not in itself settle the question of whether they are that person. Similarly, the claim that 'something' can 'claim' that it is a person does not, in itself, settle the question of whether it is a person. This is because the capacity to makes such a claim, implicitly or explicitly, may not be the only minimum condition of proper function which must be satisfied.

The lack of any straightforward classical exponents of this theory is compensated for by the very many philosophers who hold something at least very akin to this theory today. Perhaps the most influential modern exponent is Bernard Williams.

The principal insights of theory are as follows:

- Since it holds that the criteria of person and same person we actually use most of the time are the criteria we must use, the theory does full justice to the third-person perspective.
- It provides an explanation for both mental and physical concepts applying to persons.
- It is consistent with empirical data in that it explains why our ordinary concept of person should run into radical difficulties when we seek to apply it to damaged or dysfunctioning individuals.

The principal failures of the theory are as follows (see conditions (1), (2) (perhaps), (3), (4), and (5):

- The first-person perspective is made to appear irrelevant to personhood (condition (1)).

- It is not at all clear that the minimum conditions of proper function can be derived in a non-circular way (condition (2)).
- Much of the plausibility of the theory derives from the fact that it connects with our ordinary criteria of same person, i.e. same body. But, under pressure, the brain version of the theory comes to the fore and it is not clear that this could have the same connections with our ordinary ways of thinking. The theory does not allow for the possibility of non-human persons, and not all of the concepts employed are fundamental (conditions (3), (4), and (5)).

Non-normative theories

One way of thinking about the complexities of these theories is to translate their principal ideas into 'mind experiments', in which we construct a hypothetical set of events in which various things happen to us. At the end of the story, we can then ask ourselves whether we feel that the person has survived, and if so, in what sense this has happened. Conversely, we may feel that the person has not survived, and we can then start to think about why we feel this to be the case.

Philosophers have frequently devised mind experiments as ways of demonstrating the consequences of holding different views of personhood, and the scope of such experiments has gradually widened with the advent of possible technology and the growth in science fiction – many such mind experiments seem to owe more than a little to the scripts of *Star Trek* episodes. In a mind experiment, the reader is presented with a scenario in which things happen to a person, and they are asked to consider whether the person remains the same person throughout, and if so, where it is that personhood resides.

After the following three mind experiments, there is one real experiment in which the physiological mechanisms of the brain are discussed in relation to personhood.

Consider this series of events:

As George awoke one morning from uneasy dreams, concerning the iniquity of the present Government and the prospect of cruel and unusual punishments, he found himself in a rather confused state of mind. Although the bedroom did seem vaguely familiar to him, he could not quite recall where he was and what he was doing there. After a time, the confusion cleared. But not because he could now remember where he was. On the contrary. His confusion cleared only because the room ceased to look familiar at all. Indeed it now seemed to him a very bizarre room full of strange objects whose purpose he could not fathom and which induced in him a peculiar sense of anxiety. With everything else however, he was perfectly content. For whatever else happened, whether through royal pardon or else by the daring efforts of his fellow conspirators, he had at the very last moment escaped from the hangman at Tyburn. Guy Fawkes was free!

When George's family came into the room, they discovered that their dear father was acting very strangely indeed. Not only did he profess not to know them but he also claimed to know others whom he had never even mentioned before. Indeed he claimed to remember witnessing events and doing things which he had never mentioned before. So disturbed was his behaviour that his anxious and astonished family decided to call for expert help.

In the subsequent investigations, it so happened that all the events George claimed to remember witnessing and all the activities he claimed to have engaged in, pointed unanimously to the life-history of one Guy Fawkes. Not only did all the verifiable claims he made fit the pattern of Fawkes' life as known to historians, but claims that could not be checked were judged to be most plausible and to provide explanations of hitherto unexplained events. The final proof came however when he told scientists just where to find a stash of weapons and spare barrels of gunpowder. And indeed just such a stash was found buried deep in earth that had lain undisturbed for centuries. His description of one of the guns could not have been more precise. When news of this finally leaked out, the judgement of the newspapers was unequivocal. 'GUY FAWKES BACK WITH A BANG' ran the headline in *The Sun*. 'Libyan connection denied by Fawkes' said *The Telegraph*.

Williams, in discussing this scenario comments:

But newspapers are prone to exaggeration, and this might be an exaggeration . . . we are not forced to accept the description of [George's] condition as his being identical with Guy Fawkes. I shall now put forward an argument to strengthen this contention and to suggest that we should not be justified in accepting the description. If it is logically possible that [George] should undergo the changes described then it's logically possible that someone else should simultaneously undergo the same changes; e.g. that both [George] and his brother Robert should be found in this condition. What should we say in that case? They cannot both be Guy Fawkes; if they were, Guy Fawkes would be in two places at the same time which is absurd. Moreover if they were both identical with Guy Fawkes, they would be identical with each other which is also absurd. Hence we could not say that they were both identical with Guy Fawkes. We might say instead that one of them was identical with Guy Fawkes, and that the other was just like him; but this would be an utterly vacuous manoeuvre since there would *ex hypothesi* be no principle determining which description was to apply to which. So it would be best, if anything, to say that both had mysteriously become like Guy Fawkes, clairvoyantly knew about him, or something like this. If this would be the best description of each of the two, why would it not be the best description of [George] if [George] alone were changed?

With permission, Williams B. (1973)

WHERE AM I?

. . . At first I was a bit reluctant, Would it really work? The Houston brain surgeons encouraged me. 'Think of it,' they said 'as a mere stretching of the nerves. If your brain were just moved over an inch in your skull, that would not alter or impair your mind. We're simply going to make the nerves [between your brain and your body] indefinitely elastic by splicing radio links into them.

I was shown around the life support lab in Houston and saw the sparkling new vat in which my brain would be placed, were I to agree. I met the large and brilliant support team of neurologists, haematologists, biophysicists, and electrical engineers. I agreed to give it a try . . .

. . . The day for surgery arrived at last and of course I was anaesthetised and remember nothing of the operation itself. When I came out of anaesthesia, I opened my eyes, looked around, and asked the inevitable, the traditional, the lamentably hackneyed postoperative question. 'Where am I?' The nurse smiled down at me. 'You're in Houston,' she said and I reflected that this still had a good chance of being the truth one way or another. She handed me a mirror. Sure enough, there were the tiny antennae pointing up through their titanium ports cemented in to my skull.

'I gather the operation was a success,' I said. 'I want to go and see my brain.' They led me (I was a bit dizzy and unsteady) down a long corridor and into the life-support lab. A cheer went up from the assembled support team, and I responded with what I hoped was a jaunty salute. Still feeling light-headed, I was helped over to the life-support vat. I peered through the glass. There, floating in what looked like ginger ale, was undeniably a human brain, though it was almost covered with printed circuit chips, plastic tubules, electrodes and other paraphernalia. 'Is that mine?' I asked. 'Hit the output transmitter switch there on the side of the vat and see for yourself,' the project director replied. I moved the switch to OFF and immediately slumped groggy and nauseated, into the arms of the technicians, one of whom kindly restored the switch to its ON position. While I recovered my equilibrium and composure, I thought to myself: 'Well, here I am sitting on a folding chair, staring through a piece of plate glass at my own brain . . . 'But wait,' I said to myself, 'shouldn't I have thought to myself: "Well, here I am, suspended in a bubbling fluid, being stared at by my own eyes?"' I tried to think this latter thought. I tried to project it into the tank, offering it hopefully to my brain, but I failed to carry off the exercise with any conviction. I tried again. 'Here am I, Daniel Dennet, suspended in a bubbling fluid being stared at by my own eyes'. No, it just didn't work. Most puzzling and confusing. Being a philosopher of firm physicalist conviction, I believed unswervingly that the tokening of my thoughts was occurring somewhere in my brain: yet, when I thought 'Here I am' where the thought occurred was here, outside the vat, where I, Dennet, was standing staring at my brain.

I tried and tried to think myself into the vat, but to no avail. I tried to build up to the task by doing mental exercises. I thought to myself, 'The sun is shining over there' five times in succession, each time mentally ostending [= pointing] a different place: in order, the sunlit corner of the lab, the visible front lawn of the hospital, Houston, Mars and Jupiter. I found I had little difficulty in getting my 'there's' to hop all over the celestial map with their proper references. I could loft a 'there' in an instant through the farthest reaches of space and then aim the next 'there' with pinpoint accuracy at the upper left quadrant of a freckle on my arm. Why was I having such trouble with 'here'? 'Here in Houston' worked well enough and so did 'here in the lab', and even 'here in this part of the lab' but 'here in the vat' always seemed an unmeant mental mouthing. I tried closing my eyes while thinking it. This seemed to help but still I couldn't manage to pull it off except perhaps for a fleeting instant. I couldn't be sure. The discovery that I couldn' t be sure was also unsettling. How did I know where I meant by 'here' when I thought 'here'? Could I think I meant one place when in fact I meant another? Perhaps I was incorrigible about where I meant when I said 'here'. But in my present circumstances it seems that either I was doomed by sheer force of mental habit to thinking systematically false indexical thoughts or where a person is (and hence where his thoughts occur) is not necessarily where his brain, the physical seat of his soul, resides.

With permission, Dennet D.C. (1978)

WHICH AM I?

The Teletransporter

I enter the Teletransporter. I have been taken to Mars before, but only by the old method, a space ship journey taking several weeks. This machine will send me at the speed of light. I merely have to press the button. Like others I am nervous. Will it work? I remind myself what I have been told to expect. When I press the button, I shall lose consciousness, and then wake up at what seems a moment later. In fact I shall have been unconscious for about an hour. The scanner here on Earth will destroy my brain and body, while recording the exact states of all my cells. It will then transmit this information by radio. Travelling at the speed of light, the message will take three minutes to reach the Replicator on Mars. This will then create, out of new matter, a brain and a body exactly like mine. It will be in this body that I shall wake up.

Though I believe that this will happen, I still hesitate. But then I remember seeing my wife grin when, at breakfast today, I revealed my nervousness. As she reminded me, she has been often teletransported and there is nothing wrong with her. I press the button. As predicted, I lose and seem at once to regain consciousness, but in a different cubicle. Examining my new body, I find no change at all. Even the cut on my upper lip, from this morning's shave, is still there.

Several years pass, during which I am often teletransported. I am now back in the cubicle, ready for another trip to Mars. But this time, when I press the green button, I do not lose consciousness. There is a whirring sound, then silence. I leave the cubicle, and say to the attendant: 'It's not working. What did I do wrong?'

'It's working,' he replies, handing me a printed card.

Message to our Customers

The Teletransporter will now transfer you to your destination without destroying your original brain and body. We hope you will welcome the personal opportunities this technological advance affords.

TT Inc.

The attendant tells me that I am one of the first people to use the new Scanner. He adds that, if I stay for an hour, I can use the intercom to see and talk to myself on Mars.

'Wait a minute,' I reply, 'If I'm here I can't also be on Mars.'

Someone politely coughs, a white-coated man who asks to speak to me in private. We go to his office, where he tells me to sit down, and pauses. Then he says: 'I'm afraid that we're having problems with the new Scanner. It records your blueprint just as accurately, as you will see when you talk to yourself on Mars. But it seems to be damaging the cardiac systems which it scans. Judging from the results so far, though you will be quite healthy on Mars, here on Earth you must expect cardiac failure within a few days.

The attendant later calls me to the Intercom. On the screen I see myself just as I do in the mirror every morning. On the screen I am not left-right reversed. And, while I stand here speechless, I can see and hear myself, in the studio on Mars, starting to speak.

The figure on the screen tries to console me with the same thoughts with which I recently tried to console a dying friend. It is sad to learn, on the receiving end, how unconsoling these thoughts are. My replica then assures me that he will take up my life where I leave off. He loves my wife and together they will care for my children. And he will finish the book that I am writing. Besides having all my drafts, he has all of my intentions. I must admit that he can finish my book as well as I could. All these facts console me a little. Even so, I shall soon lose consciousness, forever.

With permission, Parfit, D. (1984)

HOW MANY AM I?

This is essentially a 'real experiment' in which the physiological mechanisms of the brain are discussed in relation to personhood. The author reviews the consequences of an operation on the brain which severs the higher connections between the two cerebral hemispheres, and argues that there are five possible philosophical interpretations of the results. After reading his account, and his suggested interpretations, the reader should think about their own preferred interpretation.

The brains of human beings and other mammals consist of two hemispheres, the left and the right (from the point of view of the 'owner'). Each hemisphere is associated with a set of functions. Amongst other functions, the right hemisphere is largely responsible for perceptual recognition. The left hemisphere has different functions and usually controls the production of speech. Also, by and large, the left cerebral hemisphere is associated with the right side of the body and the right hemisphere with the left side. Tactual stimuli from one side are transmitted to the opposite hemisphere – with the exception of the head and neck, which are connected to both sides. In addition, the left half of each retina, i.e. that which scans the right half of the visual field, sends impulses to the left hemisphere, and impulses from the left half of the visual field are transmitted by the right half of each retina to the right hemisphere. Auditory impulses from each ear are to some degree transmitted to both hemispheres. Smells, on the other hand, are transmitted ipsilaterally: the left nostril transmits to the left hemisphere and the right nostril to the right.

Both hemispheres are linked to the spinal column and peripheral nerves through a common brain stem, but they also communicate directly with one another, by a large transverse band of nerve fibres called the corpus callosum, plus some smaller pathways. These direct cerebral commissures play an essential role in the ordinary integration of function between the hemispheres of normal persons.

After the brain-splitting operation for epilepsy, certain phenomena have been observed when sensory stimuli are segregated to the two hemispheres.

The results are as follows. What is flashed to the right half of the visual field, or felt unseen by the right hand, can be reported verbally. What is flashed to the left half field or felt by the left hand cannot be reported, though if the word 'hat' is flashed on the left, the left hand will retrieve a hat from a group of concealed objects if the person is told to pick out what he has seen. At the same time he will insist verbally that he saw nothing. Or, if two different words are flashed to the two half fields (e.g. 'pencil' and 'toothbrush') and the individual is told to retrieve the corresponding object from beneath a screen, with both hands, then the hands will search the collection of objects independently, the right hand picking up the pencil and discarding it while the left hand searches for it, and the left hand similarly rejecting the toothbrush which the right hand lights upon with satisfaction. Again, under such conditions, if a chimeric figure composed of pictures of the faces of two people, say a young boy and a woman, is shown in such a way that each hemisphere is stimulated by only half of the picture, the person will not report anything odd about the face. However, when asked, he will describe, say, the face of a young boy. But asked to pick out the face from an array of faces he will point to that of a woman.

If a concealed object is placed in the left hand and the person is asked to guess what it is, wrong guesses will elicit an annoyed frown, since the right hemisphere, which receives the tactile information, also hears the answers. If the speaking hemisphere should guess correctly, the result is a smile. A smell fed to the right nostril (which stimulates the right hemisphere) will elicit a verbal denial that the subject smells anything, but if asked to point with the left hand at a corresponding object he will succeed in picking out, for example, a clove of garlic, protesting all the while that he smells absolutely nothing, so how can he possibly point to what he smells? If the smell is an unpleasant one like that of rotten eggs, these denials will be accompanied by wrinklings of the nose and mouth, and guttural exclamations of disgust.

One particularly poignant example of conflict between the hemispheres is as follows. A pipe is placed out of sight in the patient's left hand, and he is then asked to write with his left hand what he is holding. Very laboriously and heavily, the left hand writes the letters P and I. Then suddenly the writing speeds up and becomes lighter, the I is converted into an E, and the word is completed as PENCIL. Evidently the left hemisphere has made a guess based on the appearance of the first two letters, and has interfered with ipsilateral control. But then the right hemisphere takes over control of the hand again, heavily crosses out the letters ENCIL, and draws a crude picture of a pipe.

All this is combined with what appears to be complete normalcy in ordinary activities, when no segregation of input to the two hemispheres has been artificially created. Both sides fall asleep and wake up at the same time. The patients can play the piano, button their shirts, swim, and perform well in other activities requiring bilateral co-ordination. Moreover they do not report any sensation of division or reduction of the visual field.

Adapted from T. Nagel, with permission (1979)

There appear to be five interpretations of the experimental data which utilize the concept of an individual mind.

- The patients have one fairly normal mind associated with the left hemisphere, and the responses emanating from the non-verbal right hemisphere are the responses of an automaton, and are not produced by conscious mental processes.
- The patients have only one mind associated with the left hemisphere, but there also occur (associated with the right hemisphere) isolated conscious

mental phenomena, not integrated into a mind at all, though they can perhaps be ascribed to the organism.

- The patients have two minds, one which can talk and one which cannot.
- They have one mind, whose contents derive from both hemispheres and are rather peculiar and dissociated.
- They have one normal mind most of the time, while the hemispheres are functioning in parallel, but two minds are elicited by the experimental situations which yield the interesting results. (Perhaps the single mind splits in two and reconvenes when the experiment is over.)

Conclusion

What can be concluded from this discussion is that pinpointing the person is a contentious thing to do. If we return to the example of the patient with Alzheimer's disease, we can see that their personhood remains intact if we apply the notion of 'soul', is problematic if we apply the notion of 'experience' (because recent experiences are not recalled and therefore 'lost'), and if we apply 'body' theories, personhood is questionable because of the malfunction of the brain. These theories, therefore, disagree whether or not people in the late stages of Alzheimer's disease are persons.

What seems evident, therefore, from the theories and thought experiments we have presented in this chapter, is that the notion of being a 'person' is much more problematic than most us ordinarily think. At heart, the problem is that the notion of 'person' that we have inherited and which we use in everyday discourse, including moral discourse, is an all-or-nothing notion. That is, our notion of personhood does not admit of degrees. Something either is or is not a person. But the reality of human beings is quite different. We need to remind ourselves of this. As we have seen, in nursing we are familiar with patients who exhibit some, but not all, of the characteristics which we take to be definitive of 'personhood'.

But the problem is not confined to dysfunctional or ill human beings. Perfectly ordinary and healthy human beings are in just this condition for a significant period of their lives, namely the period which ends somewhere in childhood and begins somewhere after their conception. Neither embryos, foetuses, neonates, babies or young infants are unambiguously persons. Indeed, much of the debate about the morality of abortion seems to centre on the question of the personhood (or lack of it) of prenatal human beings. But, if it is a mistake to try and map an all-or-nothing notion of personhood onto human beings, then attempts to settle the morality of abortion by appeal to notions of personhood are doomed to fail. We may, of course, simply stipulate in law that abortion should not be carried out after a certain stage of gestation. But this does not mean that we have discovered or even decided what a person really is.

Just as we cannot believe that personhood gets switched on at a particular moment of gestation so we cannot believe that it gets switched off at a particular moment of decay or disease. Of course, persons can die and cease to be persons. But then they do so in virtue of ceasing to be living human beings.

In nursing, especially, we should not accept the assumption that one's status as a person is the engine that should drive the moral reactions and judgements of others. Even if we were able to settle the nature of person-hood, it would not follow that it should remain at the heart of moral care and respect. For this will mean that our moral respect is also likely to be all or nothing and not to admit of the degrees that characterize the real moral world. We may believe that even human beings at the remotest distances from persons, zygotes and victims of brain-stem injuries, are not to be treated in just any way we like, to be used for this or that purpose. And this not because we are oversqueamish or because we fear the slippery slope of treating real persons in the same way. Rather, we may believe these human beings are deserving of respect and of care commensurate with their natures. No one thinks we should confer the right to vote on embryos. It does not follow that they can be disposed of as mere stuff. Most of us are saddened but nevertheless relieved when our increasingly senile relatives are prevented from driving. But we do not conclude that they can now be deprived of all other rights.

In the absence of any objective conception of what it is to be a person, we are in the end thrown back upon our experience and our affective responses. It is our affective responses and not objective characteristics that must drive our moral language in this area. And in the hard cases of abortion, euthanasia and treatment of the very young and the very old and the very sick, we have to determine what feelings we are able to live with. What feelings we can make part of our own identity as citizens, relatives and health professionals. So, in the end, the question we have to face in nursing is not, 'but are they persons?' but rather 'what kind of people do we want to be?' In other words, we need to think about how we want to act towards others, rather than how those others require action from us by virtue of definitions of personhood.

It should be noted that many of the ideas in this chapter were first developed in Grand and Hughes (1996).

References

Dennett, D.C. 1978: *Brainstorms. Philosophical essays on mind and psychology.* London: Harvester.

Eccles, J. 1977: *The self and its brain.* New York: Springer.

Ground, I. and Hughes, J 1996: *Business matters.* London: Infocomm.

Hume, D. 1978: *A treatise on human nature.* Oxford: Oxford University Press.

Locke, J. 1964: *An essay concerning human understanding.* London: Collins/Fontana.

Nagel, T. 1979: *Brain bisection and the unity of consciousness.* Mortal Questions, p. 148 ff. Cambridge: Cambridge University Press.

Parfit, D. 1984: *Reasons and persons.* Oxford: Oxford University Press.

Sacks, O. 1985: *The man who mistook his wife for a hat.* London: Gerald Duckworth.

Williams, B. 1973: *Personal identity and individuation. Problems of the self.* Cambridge: Cambridge University Press.

Further reading

Blakemore, C. 1977: *Mechanisms of the mind. BBC Reith Lectures 1976.* Cambridge: Cambridge University Press.

Boden, M.A. 1987: *Artificial intelligence and natural man,* 2nd edn. London: MIT Press.

Chomsky, N. 1972: *Language and mind.* New York: Harcourt Brace Jovanovich.

Glover, J. (ed.) 1976: *The philosophy of mind.* Readings Series. Oxford: Oxford University Press.

Johnson-Laird, P.N. 1988: *The computer and the mind.* London: Collins/Fontana.

McGinn, C. 1982: *The character of mind.* Oxford: Oxford University Press.

Pratt, J.B. 1926: *Matter and spirit.* London: Macmillan.

Ryle, G. 1963: *The concept of mind.* Harmondsworth: Penguin.

Searle, J. 1989: *Minds, brains, and science. BBC Reith Lectures 1984.* Harmondsworth: Penguin.

Strawson, P.F. 1964: *Individuals: an essay in descriptive metaphysics.* London: Methuen.

Taylor, R. 1963: *Metaphysics,* 2nd edn. Princeton, NJ.: Prentice-Hall.

Teichman, J. 1974: *The mind and the soul. An introduction to the philosophy of mind.* London: Routledge.

Warnock, G.J. (ed.) 1967: *Philosophy of perception.* Oxford: Oxford University Press.

Moral philosophy

6

Introduction

In recent years, health-care ethics has been dominated by discussion of the 'big issues' of life and death: abortion and euthanasia. But many of the moral issues which nurses faces are not particular events about which single decisions must be made, but permanent features of the relationships and structures within which nurses and patients find themselves.

This chapter argues that while these 'dramatic ethics' (Seedhouse, 1988) do indeed form an important part of the moral debate in health care, the emphasis placed on them has served to obscure other ethical debates. Moreover, the context of these dramatic issues makes their examination of more relevance to those professional groups who have primary responsibility for making these decisions (usually medical staff), than to nurses who have different ethical decisions to make. This is not to say that nurses should not have discussions about these dilemmas, or have any part in the decisions made, but that concentration on this type of dilemma obscures other decisions which nurses have to make.

One approach to this problem is, of course, to focus on 'persisting ethics' (Seedhouse, 1988), or in other words the ethical principles which underpin decision-making. Focusing on persisting ethics, however, may well give rise to other problems, largely because the values and theories which underpin them are couched in abstract and absolute terms. The nature of nursing work is such that it often involves doing things which have more than one consequence, and nursing frequently involves consideration of the relative merits of these consequences rather than simple choices between one action and another. It is suggested in this chapter, therefore, that nurses also need to understand processes and ways of thinking about ethical dilemmas.

Dramatic ethics

Seedhouse (1988) used the term 'dramatic ethics' to describe the type of specific dilemma which arises in health care 'that seems to stand self-contained, in isolation from other personal or work issues'. These dilemmas include, for example, decisions about switching off life-support systems or allocating transplant organs to patients with a poor prognosis. The debates usually involve a detailed examination of the particulars of each case, as it is recognized that sweeping generalizations about intervention are out of place. The aim of the debate is very clear to those participating in the debate – a choice has to be made between courses of action, that is, the specific debate must lead to a specific conclusion.

Although dramatic ethical debates are contextual, in that they involve examination of the circumstances in which the debate has arisen, they are also 'episodic', in that they refer to particular episodes in a patient's career. In other words, they seem to be 'one-off' decisions made in specific instances, and have limited reference to the way in which care is generally given. In addition, dramatic ethics are often issues which involve consideration of the power and practices of the particular professional group which has responsibility for these decisions, and in the current structure of health care this is most often the medical profession.

There is a relationship between the type of ethical dilemma which presents to a professional group and the way in which this group practices. Doctors, for example, have an episodic contact with patients because of the way in which they work. They will see patients for periods of time which are usually devoted to the carrying out of a specific medical task. Thus patients will see doctors for diagnostic episodes or treatment episodes, for example, and when these tasks are finished, the contact ends. Nurses, on the other hand, are moving towards a much more diffuse way of working. Whereas, in the past, 'task allocation' was a common approach, where nurses would have contact with patients only to perform specific tasks, notions of holistic, patient-centred care have become more generally accepted as ideals of nursing care. This leads to more sustained contact with patients, as in the case of primary nursing, and also more diffuse interaction, where nurses will give different forms of care, often simultaneously.

The relevance of working practices to the ethical dilemmas which present to health-care workers can be illustrated by attempting to imagine how a dramatic ethical issue might present to a nurse. Firstly, we could think of a traditional dramatic issue, say for example the decision to turn off a life-support system when a patient is unconscious and showing no sign of meaningful neurological activity. The decision which the doctor makes is based on clinical indicators and on ethical principles, and the issue is whether the system should be switched off or not.

For the nurse, however, the patient presents a different set of questions. The nurse may have a part in the discussion about whether to continue treatment, but her role in the health-care organization means that she does not actually make this decision. The questions that the patient presents to the nurse are much more about the way in which this patient should be treated generally, for example whether the patient should still be respected and treated as a person, and should be talked to and handled as if aware of external events. This is the type of decision that most concerns the nurse.

Secondly, we could try to imagine what a nursing dramatic issue would be, bearing in mind the description that Seedhouse gives of a dramatic dilemma as one which 'seems to stand self-contained, in isolation from other personal or work issues'. This is extremely difficult to do. Examples of dilemmas which spring to mind might include situations like whether to tell a patient of a terminal diagnosis, whether to attempt to dissuade a patient from suicide, or perhaps whether to resuscitate a patient who is terminally ill. On further examination, however, these dilemmas are not self-contained, because they arise in the context of underlying principles of acting morally towards patients, or, in other words, in the context of the principles on which relationships with patients are based. These dilemmas are not self-contained, they are simply crises within the context of care.

It is, of course, questionable whether there are any examples of 'pure' dramatic ethics in which underlying principles play little or no part. Even the debate about switching off a ventilator involves, or should involve, some reference to the underlying principles of care. Seedhouse describes dramatic ethics as the 'tip of the iceberg', arguing that another type of ethics, which he calls 'persisting ethics' (involving the principles of care), can be thought of as part of the iceberg which is not usually visible. The point that is being made here, therefore, is that concentration on dramatic ethics serves to obscure persisting ethics and the way in which they can be brought to bear on ethical decision-making.

Persisting ethics

Seedhouse (1988: p. 21) describes persisting ethics as 'the continuing issues which constantly underlie the dramatic cases'. Persisting ethics therefore include issues such as what it means to be a person, issues about autonomy and freedom, and human rights. These are the issues which are to be found under debate in general texts on ethics, and in this sense they are a familiar part of mainstream ethical theory. The nurse who has questions about persistent ethics is therefore likely to be able to draw upon a plethora of writing about these issues.

To take an example of an issue in persisting ethics, the issue of patient freedom is one which has been extensively discussed in health-care debates. Patient freedom to make choices about their treatment affects dramatic debates about, say euthanasia, but also more mundane choices about compliance with drug regimes and even the decision whether to eat hospital food or not. We can see, therefore, that an understanding of the persistent ethics of patient freedom has wider implications than simply dramatic episodes in care.

When considering persisting ethics, the nurse has, as mentioned above, the opportunity to read many related texts in ethical literature. The issue of personal freedom, for example, has been the subject of much debate, from J.S. Mill's discussions of the limits which must be placed on intrusions on personal liberty (Himmelfarb, 1982), to existentialist discussions of the authenticity of actions which are not determined by social conventions and constraints (Warnock, 1970). This literature encompasses a wide range of positions which can be applied to health-care debates, and, importantly, debates in other areas outside health care.

A focus on persisting ethics, therefore, seems to have much to offer the nurse. It illuminates the background to dramatic ethics, and can inform practice in circumstances where ethical issues have not previously been recognized. In addition, the relationship of persisting ethics to ethical theory can extend debates beyond health care, and also give nurses insight into and experience of the processes of ethical debate.

Problems can arise, however, even when basic ethical principles have been well examined and thought through. Basic ethical principles tend to be couched in abstract terms, particularly in ethical theory. In moral philosophy, ethical theory has been historically associated with attempts to define 'the good', in other words the primary characteristics of good actions. With such a huge project it is not surprising that ethical theory has tended to be couched in abstract terms, and interpreted as absolute prescriptions for behaviour. These general statements, however, have a way of losing their power to inform practice, when nurses are faced with the messy realities of patient care. It is not often the case that a dilemma can be neatly categorized as 'being about' one issue, or even if this is the case, that general principles can help to decide particular courses of action.

The moral point of view

Ethical theory can, nevertheless, be useful in thinking about ethical debates, in the way that it provides a space in which to consider principles and their consequences. There are, however, some points which should be borne in mind when considering how to use ethical theory and conducting ethical debates.

Ethics big 'E' and small 'e'

When we first begin to think and reflect on moral matters it is easy to get distracted by two senses of ethics, between an everyday sense of this term and the term as it sometimes used by philosophers, what we might call Ethics with a capital 'E'.* Ordinarily, when we talk about the ethics (lowercase 'e') of some particular situation or of some particular person, we mean to refer to specific moral principles and ideas which govern or ought to govern that situation or that particular person's conduct. So, when say, we talk about the ethics of the prime minister, we mean to refer to the sorts of moral decision that the prime minister makes and the sorts of attitudes and ideas which lead the prime minister to make those decisions.

Now, Ethics in the philosopher's sense is a branch of philosophical inquiry like the philosophy of science or logic. It is a species of philosophical reflection. It is the name of the systematic study of the nature of our moral thinking and, simply as an intellectual inquiry, it need not involve commitment to some particular view about the things that we regard as morally right or wrong.

Now distinguishing these two senses would be a trivial matter except for the consequences of getting them mixed up. If we do mix them up, one of

---

* This convention will be used throughout this section.

two things can happen. First we might tend to think that every Ethical theory is simply a very abstract way of enshrining some particular set of views about what is morally right and wrong and therefore has no claim to being an objective intellectual inquiry. And this will tend to make us miss the role that systematic reflection about the nature of our moral thinking can play in shaping the character of the actual moral decisions that we make. Indeed, it might mislead us into thinking that moral decisions are just expressions of brute feelings and emotions.

Alternatively, mixing up these senses might lead us to think that a person's ethics must involve some commitment to some particular theory in Ethics. And this might mislead us into thinking that making ethical decisions is always and only a very intellectual business and is something in which our emotions should never be involved.

The result of mixing up these two senses of ethics then might be to blind us to the fact that in making our moral decisions, thought and feeling are both legitimately involved. In making moral decisions, we need to be compassionate, sympathetic, involved just as much as we need to be consistent, objective and detached. Indeed rather than thinking of what we morally think as something quite separable from what we morally feel, it would be better to think of our moral feelings, our compassion, sympathy and so on, but also, greed, envy and the rest – it would be better to think of these moral feelings as the inside of our moral thought. Certainly, when our hearts and our heads are out of kilter with one another, as they not infrequently are, we know that we have some hard work to do to put things right.

So, being clear about the distinction between ethics as the particular moral views which someone has, and Ethics as the systematic intellectual inquiry into the nature of such moral views in general is not just a trivial matter of semantics.

This does not mean, however, that the two senses are quite unrelated. On the contrary. First of all, philosophers can (and do) legitimately argue for particular moral views about particular moral issues. Second, and perhaps more important, the people who really matter, that is, the people who are not professional philosophers, can (and do) reflect systematically on their own personal ethics and the ethics of those around them. Insofar as any of us ever reflect on the nature of our own moral views, then we are doing Ethics.

Ethics has therefore these two related senses: one relates to the actual sorts of moral decision that some person or some person in some particular situation or role makes, whilst the other refers to that systemic reflection about the nature of those moral decisions. Of course, this is not much good unless we have some account of what kind of decision a moral decision is.

The first and philosophically most fundamental question is this: what is a moral problem or a moral judgement? What is it, if anything, that distinguishes a moral question from, say one of fact, or of taste, or of law or prudence? We can perhaps see right away that we are using 'moral' here not in opposition to 'immoral', but in opposition to 'non-moral'. It is important to point this out because over the last century or so, the term 'moral' has come to acquire a number of parasitic uses that are too often mistaken for the host meaning. Thus, in one sense, commonly used by newspapers, the term 'moral' has come to refer almost exclusively to the sexual activities of the clergy and/or prominent members of government. How this has happened is rather complicated. It seems that morality has become identified with a set of injunctions concerning one aspect of life – sexuality – which, it so happens, are particularly difficult or interesting to comply with. Another parasitic use of 'moral' has a pejorative or disparaging sense. Thus when one writer complained that he 'knew of no spectacle so ridiculous as the British people in one of its periodical fits of morality', the complaint is not that people are suddenly wondering what they ought to do but that, once again, they are behaving like hypocrites. And this itself is, of course, a moral criticism. But this use of moral parallels the history of many other words in the language. A term which is incessantly used for insincerely or doubtfully praising others can easily end up being used to express sincere and certain dislike.

Yet another common use of 'moral' is in the context of the uneasy opposition between the private, inner or personal life and the communal historically conditioned public life. Thus morality comes to be seen as an artificial set of injunctions against which the individual has to struggle. It is in this context that the amoralist can come to seem like some kind of macho hero, one against the herd. Like the other parasitic uses of 'morality', this use can come to cause philosophical difficulties in the way we talk about moral matters. For the false opposition between the supposed naturally solitary life of the real individual and the artificial social individual can lead us onto blatant but peculiarly insidious confusion and contradiction, It is this use of 'moral' which is part of what causes people to say such things as 'It's always wrong to make moral judgements' or even 'You ought not to make moral judgements' (Midgley, 1981).

One final parasitic use of 'moral' which is of particular relevance to health-care ethics is this: very often, 'moral' is used to distinguish a particular kind of point of view on something as opposed to some other possible kind of point of view. Thus one may hear politicians arguing that 'Certainly from a moral point of view, it would be desirable to expand this aspect of the health service but from an economic point of view, it would not represent value for money'. Or again, from the moral point of view, 'I ought to tell my patient about this but as a doctor . . .' In this way, the moral point of view comes to be seen as just one amongst a group of competing points of view – the political, the economic, the professional, the medical, the scientific, the aesthetic, the emotional, the administrative, and so on. But while there may be some point in contrasting the moral with the factual or the economic and the legal, and so on, this way of thinking can lead us into real difficulty. The difficulty arises because so many of the ways in which we understand the world have become just one 'point of view' amongst others that we have been left with no way of understanding the clashes between them and no way of resolving such conflicts. If the moral is just one point of view amongst others, how are we to decide which point of view we *ought* to give preference to in this particular case? A poorly sighted man cannot compare differently tinted spectacles, without actually trying some on. But which pair he puts on will affect the way he sees the other pairs.

There are two ways out of this dilemma. The first is to appeal to the existence of some neutral supreme authority. Traditionally, the prime candidate of this post has been our capacity for reason. Thus reason is often regarded as impersonal, neutral, omnicompetent – something on quite a different plane from all other competing points of view. This is as if our fellow with the spectacles were to ask the optician for his view, treating it as decisive and binding. Thus, which point of view it is proper to adopt in any given situation is the one it is most rational to adopt. But almost as soon as we say this, we can see that this is not really a way of the problem at all. For the model of reason we are using here is really a mythological one – a kind of cross between a chief administrator and Mr Spock from *Star Trek*. Rationality is amongst other things, a capacity for giving reasons for judgements, actions, decisions, and so on. But what kind of reason can we give here without prejudicing the issue of which point of view we are to take up? To return to our analogy; the optician has no preferences about which kind of tint the customer should wear. So if we are to think of the moral point of view as just one amongst others, all with equal status, we cannot simply appeal to reason to sort out the conflicts. Reason can only begin to operate once we have secured one point of view on the issue at stake.

The way out of the problem is to deny that the moral point of view is one on the same level as the political, the economic, the aesthetic and the rest. We need to be reminded that moral thinking is not simply one set of priorities but the primary way in which we sort out priorities, whether they be political, medical or economic. It is not like our mythological conception of reason, uselessly neutral, but that does not mean that it is therefore hopelessly biased. For if it is, we shall be unable to give an account of what is wrong with being biased in this respect. So one of the things we can see when we think about this question of what distinguishes the moral from the non-moral, then, is that we often need to be reminded that our actual use of moral concepts is much wider that we often think it to be. It is not as we believe it to be, one set of special considerations amongst all the rest. It is rather constitutive of our capacity for recognizing and distinguishing between different points of view. Morality is not just another pair of tinted spectacles. It is part of vision itself.

Ethical theories

Having considered the nature of moral philosophy, it is useful here to outline some important ethical theories and to get a more detailed understanding of what forms they can take, and what issues they address. We have chosen to concentrate on two major theories: utilitarianism, which concentrates on the outcome of actions, and deontology, which can be described as concentrating on the intention behind actions. The synopsis of these theories is necessarily brief, but it gives some idea of the range and scope of ethical theory.

Utilitarianism

Utilitarianism can be understood as a movement for legal, political and social reform that flourished in the nineteenth century or, again, as the ideology of that movement. But it is perhaps best understood today as a moral theory which attempts to provide a criterion for distinguishing between right and wrong actions. However, utilitarianism is nothing if not ambitious and its proponents seek to do two things by proposing this criterion. First of all they wish to explain the nature of morality and goodness. This, of course, is an objective of any ethical theory: to understand what we are doing when we make moral decisions, judgements and commitments and second to understand why it matters that we get this right; to understand the point of morality.

Unlike many other philosophical theories of morality, however, utilitarians are far from content with succeeding in reaching this intellectual goal. For, as they see it, the point of this explanation and understanding is not just the sort of point that any good philosophical explanation has. (Whatever that might be.) It is actually to try and make the world a better place to live in. And for the most part they think that the main reason why the world is not the place it ought to be is not a matter of will. It is a matter of understanding. People do not have the resources to see clearly enough what they ought to do and why they ought to do it. They do not understand morality. And the reason they do not understand it is because morality is in a mess. For the utilitarian, morality can seem like a psychopathic traffic cop on an otherwise empty highway – demanding that we go in two directions at the same time in order to avoid obstacles that would not otherwise be there.

Utilitarians, therefore, are utterly committed to reforming what they see as ordinary or traditional morality by making it more rational, systematic and practical. In particular, utilitarians are often anxious to rid morality of what they see as the irrational superstitions and inconsistencies which have arisen because of the influence of religious beliefs. And the urge to replace what they see as fundamentally magical morality with a fundamentally rational morality is the global ambition of the typical utilitarian. The project is huge but so are the resources of reason.

Utilitarianism can be characterized in terms of the combination of previously but separately championed principles:

• The consequentialist principle

The rightness or wrongness of action is determined by the goodness or badness of the results that flow from it.

- The hedonist principle

  The only good thing in itself is pleasure and the only bad thing in itself is pain.

Given some further arguments connecting the concepts of pain and pleasure with the concept of happiness, or at least with the concept of people's judgements about their own happiness, these two principles combine to form another:

- The greatest happiness principle

  The rightness of an action is determined by the extent to which it promotes the greatest happiness of the greatest number.

As John Stuart Mill, with Jeremy Bentham the founder of classical utilitarianism, writes:

> The creed which accepts as the foundation of morals Utility or the Greatest Happiness Principle, holds that actions are right in proportion as they tend to promote happiness, wrong as they tend to produce the reverse of happiness. By happiness is intended pleasure and the absence of pain, by unhappiness, pain and the privation of pleasure.

Though both the consequentialist and the hedonist principles are separately employed in ancient philosophy and though there are a number of eighteenth century precursors, especially Cumberland, Hutchinson and Hume, it is only with Bentham that utilitarianism becomes recognizable as a distinct doctrine. Anxious to deny that contemporary social practice, especially those related to punishment, could be justified either by tradition or by divine will, Bentham puts forward the principle of utility supremely confident that any opposition is either befuddled or sinister. It is Bentham who invents the 'hedonic calculus', measuring the amount of happiness in terms of seven variables: Intensity, Duration, Certainty, Propinquity (nearness in time), Fecundity (tendency to give rise to more of the same), Purity (tendency to give rise to the contrary) and Extent (number of sentient beings affected). He goes on to invent increasingly baroque sets of classifications of the various types of pleasures and pains.

It was John Stuart Mill, however, who gave utilitarianism real philosophical credibility. In part because of the fact that his utilitarian upbringing had driven him to a nervous breakdown in his early twenties but also because he was simply a much more subtle philosopher, Mill does much to meet halfway the objections to Benthamite orthodoxy. He enriches the utilitarian concept of happiness, emphasizes the roots of the principle of utility in conscience and fellow feeling and even tries a direct 'proof' of the principle of utility itself. The result of this was a heretical deviation that eventually took over from the stricter canons of Benthamite utilitarianism. It is in Mill that we find the first real suggestion that utilitarianism must attempt a compromise with ordinary morality, through the utility of moral rules and principles, and in fact Mill came to regard liberty as having much the same fundamental importance as utility itself. Utilitarians today still have to locate themselves in a landscape of thought in which Mill's views and the more extreme Benthamite account are the main reference points.

What, then, are the principal advantages of utilitarianism as a moral theory? First of all, utilitarianism is non-transcendental (at least by its own lights); that is, it makes no appeal to anything outside human life. It thus aids in freeing morality of Christianity, in particular, and in general rids morality of all attempts to justify current practice by reference to something other than what actually happens in the real world to real people.

Second, and tied to the non-transcendental character of utilitarianism, is the idea that if utilitarianism is true then all moral issues are ultimately empirical issues. Moral questions may still be difficult, but they are no longer mysterious. Taking the mystery out of morality is an important part of what the utilitarian sees as the global elimination of excuses for acting badly.

Third, relative to other ethical and moral theories, many of the basic concepts of utilitarianism – consequentialism, happiness, empirical calculation – are minimally problematic. Certainly there are problems about what these concepts are being used to do but the concepts themselves are relatively straightforward. If there are any problems about, say, the idea of a consequence of an action, they are often problems that arise quite generally about this notion and therefore have no force against utilitarianism in particular.

Fourth, utilitarianism provides a common currency of moral thought. All disagreements can be couched in terms of empirical disagreements about what in fact will produce the most utility, that is, the greatest happiness. For even if there are non-utilitarians in the world with different and irreconcilable moral beliefs, one can calculate the comparative utility of actions recommended by each system. Utilitarianism unifies. Ultimately, the community of moral agents is identical with the community of mutually intelligible beings.

Fifth, utilitarianism says that if an action makes the best possible contribution to the general happiness that in present circumstances can be made, then it is right. This has at least two important implications. First of all, it means that we are entitled to be domestically optimistic: there is always something definitely right one can actually do. Secondly, since there cannot be an action which is both the best possible and which is also wrong, we can be cosmically optimistic. Which is to say, as Williams points out, that for utilitarianism, tragedy is always illusory; the moral universe is not stacked against us from the start.

According to utilitarianism, then, the human alone does not only suffice; it can also prosper. All in all, by its own lights, utilitarianism does not merely recommend happiness as the criterion of right action. Whilst the iniquities of the outer world may demand action, and though he would be unlikely to applaud the use of such an expression, the truth is that the utilitarian has a happy soul.

Despite this, however, there are many philosophers who do not simply think that utilitarianism is wrong, simplistic or overambitious. Many of them think that utilitarianism is not just a travesty of morality but that it is fundamentally wicked. The philosopher Elizabeth Anscombe refused to argue with anyone who thought in a utilitarian way, believing that utilitarianism was evidence of a corrupt mind. And another philosopher Bernard Williams looks forward to the day 'when we shall hear no more' of utilitarianism.

Historically, there have been three phases of objections to utilitarianism. The first phase of objections amounted to the claim that utilitarianism was vulgar and degrading. In making pleasure the end of life, it recommended a life of decadence and voluptuousness. Whatever his other views, John Stuart Mill was too much a Victorian not to be sensitive to such a charge and did much to enrich the rather narrow and simplistic calculus of pleasure and happiness he inherited from Bentham. Mill thought of higher pleasures not so much as intellectual, as just active, and could be said to have put paid to the idea that what is wrong with utilitarianism is that happiness is somehow an unanalysable or unattainable state:

Happiness . . . is not a life of rapture; but moments of such, in an existence made up of few and transitory pains, many and various pleasures, with a decided predominance of the active over the passive, and having as the foundation of the whole, not to expect more from life than it is capable of bestowing. A life thus composed, to those who have been fortunate enough to obtain it, has always appeared worthy of the name of happiness.

The second phase of objections is thought by many philosophers to have been originated by G.E. Moore and is the claim that in moving from the fact that we do pursue happiness to the fact that we ought to pursue happiness, utilitarianism commits the so-called 'naturalistic fallacy'. This is supposed by these 'non-naturalist' philosophers to be the attempt to derive an 'ought' from an 'is', an action-guiding imperative statement from a descriptive one, a value from a fact. Actually, all these are completely different ideas and none has anything to do with Moore's naturalistic fallacy. In this context it is worth noting a remark by Stanley Cavell, that the reason it is impossible to get from 'facts' to 'values' is akin to the reason it is impossible to 'get' from Paris to France. It is impossible but that does not mean that there is any problem about getting there.

In any case, as J.J.C. Smart demonstrates, utilitarianism is perfectly consistent with the view that there is such a gulf between 'is' and 'ought'. If non-naturalists are right and morality is fundamentally a matter, not of describing anything, but of making commitments and issuing imperatives, then there seems no reason why these cannot be utilitarian commitments and utilitarian imperatives.

The third phase of objections to utilitarianism, which brings us more or less to the present, has centred on the claim that if utilitarianism is correct, then our present non-utilitarian ways of going on are not just confused or incomplete but are actually unintelligible. Attention has centred particularly on the supposed inability of utilitarianism to make any sense at all of ideas of justice and of integrity. This last has focused attention on the idea of the utilitarian agent. The claim here is that utilitarianism, with its view that one may at any time be obliged to commit what would otherwise be the most appalling acts in order to avert a worse result now, is inconsistent with any idea of moral agency, of acting for oneself, that we can make intelligible to ourselves.

It is worth noting at this point that one popular objection to utilitarianism is certainly wrong. Many people's initial reaction to utilitarianism is to complain that no one can possibly know all the consequences of which their action is the cause. Like buses, causes always come in bunches and consequences spread out indefinitely into the future. How, then, can utilitarianism claim to be practical and decisive?

These claims are true but misconceived. Their proponents have failed to realize that just because utilitarianism claims to provide a practical criterion for action, both past causes and future actual consequences are irrelevant.

We need to distinguish three sorts of consequences:

- The consequences the action actually has (*absolutely right action*).
- The consequences the agent expects the action to have (*subjectively right action*).
- The consequences it is rational for the agent to expect the action to have (*objectively right action*).

To see this, suppose that this is now the last quarter of the nineteenth century, and that you see a young boy drowning, who, because you now rescue him, will be able in the future to take the name of Adolf Hitler. Learning about this, people in the future will say that it would have been fortunate indeed if you had left him to drown. The consequences your action actually had diminished overall happiness. But clearly what people will in the future be able to say is irrelevant. You must decide now and you do not know what the actual consequences of your action will be in the way in which those in the future will know. You have to predict as best you can what the consequences will be. Of course you may believe that you must rescue the boy because he has in fact fallen to Earth from the planet Venus and has brought with him the means to put an end to suffering. If so, these are the consequences you expect the action will have. But assuming you are not completely mad, you should want the consequences you expect your action to have to be identical with the consequences it would, in the light of available evidence, be rational to believe your action will have. And it is in terms of these consequences, the consequences it is at the time rational to believe the action will have, that your decisions must be judged. And clearly, the further your thoughts probe into the future, the less evidence you have and so the more rational it is to ignore far future consequences.

Scepticism about our ability to predict the consequences of our actions does not look as if it will lose the utilitarian much sleep. Compare this with a more serious, if perhaps still not conclusive, problem for utilitarianism. Benthamite utilitarianism is what we now think of as act-utilitarianism. It says that an action is right insofar as it maximizes utility. If it would maximize happiness if I broke the promise I made to you on your death bed to give your money to the cat's home rather than the hospice who need it, then so be it. But if someone, who is not a utilitarian hears about this, he may not realize how this situation differs from others where I, a good utilitarian, would keep promises. And so he might go round breaking promises even when it did not maximize happiness. Clearly, if by breaking my promise to you now, I undermine promise-keeping in general, this may outweigh the benefit to the hospice and so it would be the wrong thing to do. Also, if I always stick to my promises no matter what, then I save the time of calculating consequences. Hence there is a utility attached to abiding by principles. This way lies rule-utilitarianism which says that an action is right insofar as it belongs to a class of acts (described by the rules of an accepted practice) which maximize utility.

(Another, different reason for adopting rule-utilitarianism is that if I am to compare one action with another, I must have an idea of the sort of consequences that possible but unperformed actions might have. But the only evidence here is the consequences that action of this type had in the past and this means that I must anyway take into account the consequences of types of action and here again, existing, moral rules will be a great help.)

The more we take this line, however, the more we seem forced to abandon the reforming zeal of traditional utilitarianism. We have compromised with magical morality. What do we, as utilitarians, gain for this sacrifice? Arguably, only the problem of justifying our acceptance of the content of the moral principles of traditional morality whilst at the same time being completely incapable of regarding these as principles which have any value for their own sake. They are just rules – like driving on the left of the road.

Though this needs to be argued, however, it is far from clear that moral principles can be regarded as rules in this way. The utilitarian must now face the issue described in a different context by Peter Winch (1968):

> Morality we are told is a guide which helps [us] round [our] difficulties. But were it not for morality there would be no difficulty! This is a strange sort of guide which first puts obstacles in our path and then shows us the way round them, Would it not be far simpler and more rational to be shot of the thing altogether? Then we get on with the matter in hand, whatever it is.

Deontology

A very different set of ethical principles is offered by deontological theories, where the focus is not on the consequences of actions but on the nature of the actions themselves. The essence of deontological theories is to claim that there are some things that we must or, more often, must not do whatever the consequences of this may be.

The term 'deontology' means the study of duty. This is a term that sits uneasily in the modern mind. Many people feel rather uncomfortable talking about so and so's having a duty to do something. It seems rather old fashioned and stuffy. Interestingly, we usually do not mind using the term in connection with the work of professionals. It is clear that doctors, nurses, lawyers, teachers, and so on, all have professional duties – that is, they have standards they must observe no matter what the benefits to themselves or indeed their client from failing to conform to them: there are actions that they are absolutely obliged to carry out or absolutely prohibited from doing.

Different deontological theories may lay down different particular prohibitions, for example, the Ten Commandments. Perhaps not all of us can go along with all the Ten Commandments, but many of us are likely to have sympathy with at least some absolute prohibitions. Most of us think that there are some things that it is always wrong to do. Torturing children is wrong no matter what good might happen to come of it. Perhaps we feel able to generalize this prohibition. It is always wrong to deliberately inflict suffering on the innocent and the vulnerable. Some of these prohibitions become codified. National constitutions and international agreements often use a deontological style of expression to ban certain practices or to insist that states act in certain ways. Lists of human rights – obligations owed to people simply in virtue of their being human beings, and which cannot be overruled – are precisely deontological notions.

The obvious questions to ask about this approach are: what standards and who says so? Historically, this deontological view of moral matters has been associated with external authorities or authoritative texts. The Christian Church, the state, the Koran, the Bible, the party, the United Nations have all been sources of deontological principles. It seems to some people that because of this, deontological thinking is doomed. For, it is argued, we no longer do, or no longer are able to, take such external authorities seriously. We want to know why we should do as they say.

Against this, Kant argued that deontological prohibitions need not stem from external authority. He tried to show that moral demands like respect for other persons arise from within: in fact from our nature as rational beings. Doing things because they fit in with our preferences, or because we gain satisfaction from them, according to Kant is not a basis for moral action, simply because these inclinations are ephemeral and inconsistent. The achievement of satisfaction or pleasure as a reason for action is also suspect – doing things even though they give us no satisfaction, or may even cause us harm, is a more disinterested stance, and therefore, according to Kant, a more sound basis for morality.

In today's society, where appeals to our good nature often carry with them an implicit promise of reward, the idea of doing things simply because our reason has told us they are right, rather than for emotional satisfaction, has become an uncomfortable concept. Perhaps this is due to our life in a culture which reverences the self as the arbiter of good and the object of our existence. To follow deontological morality is, to some extent, to subsume the self to the welfare of others, and furthermore to the authority of others.

Differences between the utilitarian and deontological theories

The differences between these two theories appear unreconcilable, not necessarily in their outcome, but in their justification and evaluation of moral action. While a utilitarian might argue that a person with a serious and expensive-to-treat health problem may have to forego treatment in the interests of others, a deontologist might well argue that duties of care demand that the person receive treatment. In practice, however, moral decisions are more usually an amalgam of the two perspectives. Utilitarian decisions about resources and health services are at least partly based on deontological notions of the duties required from such services, and the notion of the greatest happiness encompasses ideas of respect for persons which often form part of deontological theories. Similarly, deontological theories can be justified in terms of the general good to be achieved by their observance. In our moral decisions we quite often incorporate ideas of the particular and the general good, weighing the balance between them.

This type of balancing act is a response to the weaknesses and strengths inherent in the extreme forms of the theories. Fixing our sights on the greatest happiness, while ignoring the suffering under our noses, can be appropriate in certain circumstances, but it is not comfortable. Similarly, ignoring the general implications and effects of our actions in favour of immediate problems can seem short-sighted and partial.

Conclusion

Applying these types of ethical theory directly to the dilemmas faced by nurses is a difficult thing to do because of the complexity of the way in which nurses work. A frequent dilemma faced by nurses is that there is no one course of action which can be regarded as universally 'good' by any criteria. This is often because nurses work in ways which are determined by resource constraints – they are constantly balancing the needs of different patients and what may help one patient may adversely affect another. Where nurses have only one patient to care for, then the problem of competing patient needs is reduced, but this still does not always simplify decision-making. This is because of the essential complexity of health-care itself, where actions are rarely unequivocal.

This point becomes more apparent when we consider the notion of holism which informs much of current thinking about nursing. Rather than reducing patients to constitutive physiological systems, or disease processes, holism exhorts us to treat the patient as a whole, and to recognize the relationship between social, physiological and psychological aspects of life. We are, therefore, aware that intervention in one of these areas may well affect others.

Nurses are, therefore, obliged to consider the results of their actions on the whole of the patient. The way that an injection is given, for example, can affect more than the patient's physiology – it can affect their psychology too in the way that they become more or less anxious about treatment. Even if consideration is given only to one aspect of care, and in general nursing this would usually be the physiological, the whole of the aspect or system is part of this consideration. Giving a powerful analgesic to a terminally ill patient, for example, not only hopefully controls pain, but it can have an impact on other aspects of physiology, perhaps respiratory function, and as such can shorten the patient's life.

These 'micro-debates' are engendered by the pragmatics of care, but they are not simply pragmatic debates – they also extend to, and incorporate, debate about persisting ethics or values. In the example of a patient being given analgesia which may effectively shorten his or her life, for example, this is not simply a debate about choice of drug, but can also be cast as one about the principles of doing good (controlling pain) and preserving life and not doing harm (creating respiratory problems). In situations like this, although the general principles might be well understood, their application to health-care dilemmas is far from straightforward.

Nursing questions about the 'right' thing to do, therefore, require more detailed discussion than simply references to the often abstract debates of ethical theories and values. Where actions have more than one consequence, and we would argue that this is the case in many nursing dilemmas, appealing to principles alone is likely only to reveal a conflict between principles, and unlikely to provide guidance towards resolving conflict. The juggling of perspectives is, therefore, inherent in nursing.

This is not to say that nursing is unique in having these difficulties; many other areas of human life demonstrate the same problems. It can be argued, however, that because of its objects of concern (human beings in need) nursing shows the shape of our moral thinking more clearly. The seemingly endless debates we may have about how to discipline children, whether to tell colleagues the truth about their work, or whether football hooligans should be imprisoned, can remain as debates for many of us. Where nursing is concerned, however, the image of the ill or suffering patient sharpens up ethical issues.

It is a mistake, however, to think that the 'moral high ground' is both unreachable and inhospitable with enough room only for a few lucky dreamers and that there is something wrong in trying to occupy it. Actually we live there all the time. (There is nowhere else to go.) Instead we may think about the use of ethical theories in the following ways:

- Moral thinking is not a matter of applying moral theories. It is a matter of seeing the world correctly. But this requires moral vocabulary. The role of theory is to supply that vocabulary.
- Moral thinking is about negotiating our way around the myriad different points of view.
- Moral thinking is not an optional extra but standard fittings for human life.

Thus we can see ethical theory as a way of thinking rather than supplying ready-made conclusions to our thought.

References

Cavell, S. 1979: *The claim of reason: Wittgenstein, skepticism, morality and tragedy.* p. 323. Oxford: Clarendon Press.

Himmelfarb, H. (ed.) 1982: *J.S. Mill. On liberty.* Harmondsworth: Penguin.

Midgley, M. 1981: *Heart & Mind.* London: Methuen.

Seedhouse, D. 1988: *Ethics: the heart of health care.* Chichester: John Wiley.

Warnock, M. 1970: *Existentialism.* Oxford: Oxford University Press.

Winch, P. 1968: *Moral integrity.* Oxford: Blackwell.

Further reading

Acton, H.B. 1970: *Kant's moral philosophy.* London: Macmillan.

Anscombe, G.E.M. 1963: *Intentions,* 2nd edn. London: Blackwell.

Aristotle 1980: *The Nicomachean Ethics.* Oxford: Oxford University Press.

Bretall, R. (ed.) 1938: *A Kierkegaard anthology.* Princeton, NJ: Princeton University Press.

Foot, P. (ed.) 1967: *Theories of ethics.* Oxford: Oxford University Press.

Frankena, W.K. 1963: *Ethics.* Englewood Cliffs, NJ: Prentice-Hall.

Frazer, E., Hornsby, J. and Lovibond, S. 1992: *Ethics: a feminist reader.* Oxford: Blackwell.

Glover, J. 1988: *Causing death and saving lives.* London: Penguin.

Hare, R.M. 1952: *The language of morals.* Oxford: Oxford University Press.

Humphreys, C. 1951: *Buddhism.* Harmondsworth: Penguin.

MacIntyre, A. 1966: *A short history of ethics.* London: Routledge and Kegan Paul.

Marcuse, H. 1972: *One dimensional man.* London: Abacus.

Midgley, M. 1978: *Beast & man.* London: Methuen.

Midgley, M. and Hughes, J. 1983: *Women's choices.* London: Wiedenfeld and Nicolson.

Moore, G.E. 1903: *Principia Ethica.* Cambridge: Cambridge University Press.

Nietzsche, F. 1973: *Beyond good and evil.* Harmondsworth: Penguin.

Paton, H.J. 1948: *The moral law.* London: Hutchinson University Press.

Paton, H.R. (trans.) 1948: *Kant. Groundwork of the metaphysics of morals.* London: Hutchinson.

Plato 1954: *The last days of Socrates.* Harmondsworth: Penguin.

Sartre, J.P. 1973: *Existentialism and humanism.* London: Methuen.

Smart, J.J.C. and Williams, B. 1973: *Utilitarianism: for and against.* Cambridge: Cambridge University Press.

Spinoza, B. 1955: *On the improvement of the understanding.* New York: Dover.

Thomson, J.A.K. (trans.) 1976: *Aristotle. Ethics.* London: Penguin.

Thompson, J. 1974: *Kierkegaard.* London: Victor Gollancz.

Warnock, M. 1960: *Ethics since 1900.* Oxford: Oxford University Press.

Warnock, M. (ed.) 1962: *Utilitarianism.* Glasgow: Fontana.

Warnock, M. 1984: *Report of the Committee of Inquiry into Human Fertilisation and Embryology.* London: HMSO.

Williams, B. 1972: *Morality: an introduction to ethics.* Cambridge: Cambridge University Press.

7

Political philosophy

Introduction

As health care becomes more and more prominent in political debate, nurses have found themselves (sometimes unwillingly) having to recognize that what they do has a political as well as a personal dimension. This is, perhaps, most apparent at a 'macro-political' level, where arguments range about the funding of health care and the duties of governments to provide services. Here the debates are about issues such as rights, duties, fairness and need, and most commonly involve positions in which health care is seen as a right which it is the duty of the state to provide, and positions which describe health care as a commodity which can be purchased, ideally without too much interference from the state which can stifle freedom and choice.

What nurses do for their patients, therefore, is to a large extent determined by the resources and structures chosen by politicians. Political choices, however, not only affect the broad structure of health-care services, but also affect the 'micro-political' issues which nurses face at the point of delivering care to patients and clients. Given that nurses frequently care for groups of patients, this caring often involves prioritizing of care, and juggling the various needs of individuals in relation to others needing care. One way of looking at this is to argue that the same issues which arise in macro-political debates are found in the decisions which nurse have to make in their daily practice.

To take an example, let us imagine that a nurse is running a child-care clinic at which she will provide advice to parents from a range of different social backgrounds. The time allotted to each client is ten minutes, and the clinic is fully booked. The first client, however, has a number of health problems, and also very difficult social circumstances – she is a single mother, with very little money, poor housing and has had little education. Her baby is suffering from asthma and bronchitis, and she will need extensive educational input to help her to care for him, in addition to support for her attempts to get better housing. This session will clearly take more than ten minutes, and it is likely that she will need more sessions in the future. To give her the time that she needs, however, will either involve reducing the time available for other clients, or extending the clinic hours, something which will inconvenience other clients by keeping them waiting and the nurse by lengthening her working day.

The number of clients that the nurse has in her clinic is largely determined by the political decisions which have been made about the need and purpose of the clinic, and the resources allocated to it, but the nurse has an immediate decision to make about how she can work within these constraints. Does she give her first client all the time that she needs, thus reducing the time available to others but recognizing differences in need, or does she try to spend exactly the same time with this client as with others, thus ensuring an equal distribution of her time, but running the risk of not adequately tackling the issues which she is supposed to address?

The way in which the nurse makes her decision will depend on many things. Her experience of running the clinic may well tell her that many of the clients will take less time than that allotted to them, and so it will be possible to manage the occasional client who needs more time. On the other hand, she may worry that those waiting will complain about her inefficiency if they are delayed too much. The quality of the relationship that she has with her first client may also affect her decision – if the woman is aggressive, she may try to hurry her along, but if she likes the woman she may feel inclined to spend more time with her.

Somewhere in all of this, however, the nurse will also be engaged in a philosophical debate: she will either be weighing up the merits of different philosophical arguments about justice, rights and duties, or she will be acting on principles which can be traced back to philosophical arguments. It is likely, however, that the nurse will not recognize her debate as being philosophical, but will instead think of it as a debate about beliefs and feelings. This is not necessarily a bad thing, as any abstract conception, such as justice, needs to have some resonance with those who apply it, and this resonance may well feel like a belief or some form of emotional affirmation. The problem is, however, that without access to, or understanding of, the context in which concepts have been developed and challenged, these principles are difficult to examine critically, and can easily become rigid dogma.

This chapter, therefore, gives an overview of political philosophy, concentrating on the areas which are of particular relevance to nursing and health care. There is some overlap between political philosophy and moral philosophy – the former is largely about the best way to organize social life and the latter is about the best way to lead our personal life, and the two lives can never be completely divorced. Our emphasis in this chapter, however, will be on the main questions raised by political philosophy, about rights, duties, justice, freedom and the like, and how these relate to both macro and micro decisions in nursing and health care.

What is political philosophy?

Drawing a boundary around political philosophy, and differentiating it from other areas of study is a difficult task, perhaps because politics has such a pervasive effect on many other areas of life, and indeed is affected by so many concerns. One obvious area of overlap is with moral philosophy – if this is seen as the search for the good life, then surely political philosophy is simply this search writ large; in other words, is political philosophy simply moral philosophy applied to the state rather than the individual? While there are some similarities between the two fields, the answer to this question has to be no, mainly because political philosophy is based on the argument that a state is a very different sort of thing to an individual person. Hegel (1956), for example, argued that the state was a distinct entity, which had an existence independent of the individuals which comprised it, and indeed, was more important and permanent than those individuals. This reification of the state, however, has been criticized by those who argue that the state is simply a convenient creation of individuals, a mechanism for organizing society which is constructed and changed by its members. Nevertheless, even if the glorification of the state is rejected (which seems to be a sensible position), there still remains a difference between arguments about how it should be constructed, and debates about the personal conduct of those who construct and comprise it. Both types of debate are about values, and both are about the best way to do things, but their subject matter, although connected, is sufficiently different in emphasis to warrant distinct examination.

Philosophical debates about political issues have a long history. Much of the work of the early Greek philosophers was concerned with determining the best way for people to be governed, and some of these early ideas are still referred to in current debates. This strong interest can be partly attributed to the situation in which the philosophers were trying to do philosophy; at the time of Socrates and Plato, Greek society was facing many problems with warring between Greek states and political conflict within them, and so it is not surprising that philosophers sought to develop some solutions to these conflicts. It is, therefore, also not surprising that 'classical' political philosophy tended to be concerned with developing ideas about the perfect society, an ambitious endeavour which has had great influence on political philosophy ever since. The search for Utopia is evident not only in the works of philosophers, but in the works of artists and writers – authors as various as More, Swift and Butler have sought to describe ideal systems of government. As centrally planned states became more imminent, however, in more recent times there have been many anti-utopian ideas evident in political debate and literature: Huxley's *Brave New World* and Orwell's *1984* are perhaps the most striking. Modern political philosophy, then, concentrates on the philosophical analysis of current systems of government rather than the attempt to define the perfect society. As politics and societies change, so does political philosophy.

At the basis of political philosophies, both modern and classic, is an idea about the nature of man. This can be implicit, as in much of the modern work, or it can be more explicit, as in, say, the work of Rousseau and Hobbes. Rousseau's notion of the nature of man was essentially a romantic and idealized one, in which he proposed that 'natural man' was a creature of good and simple ideas, who was corrupted by civilization. His political philosophy, therefore, sought to set out principles by which the state's corruptive potential could be limited and restricted, and the natural feelings of people (which were, in their natural state, good) could become the driving force of government. His book *The social contract*, written in 1762, lays forth the fundamental arguments for democracy. An earlier writer, Hobbes, on the other hand, took a much more cynical (although some would say realistic) view of human nature – that it is essentially selfish and chaotic. For this reason, he argued that people needed strong control if society was to survive. Because human life without this control would be 'solitary, poor, nasty, brutish, and short' it would be to the advantage of individuals if they accepted this control, which would regulate and improve their lives (see Hobbes, 1972).

Whatever the positions taken by philosophers about the nature of the state, or the nature of people, there are some basic concerns of political philosophy which are evident throughout their debates, and it is by looking at these concerns that the business and nature of political philosophy becomes clearer.

One way to discuss these concerns is to use the notion of state power to divide them up under the headings of authority, the justification for and nature of state power, liberty, the limits of this power, and justice, the exercise of this power. This is a broad system of classification, which in some ways is rather crude, but it does have the virtue of simplicity.

Authority

The most central task of the state is to regulate and control social life. This may be minimally according to Mill and Rousseau, or perhaps more rigorously according to Hobbes, but it is still the defining characteristic of a state. This, however, calls into question the justifications made for state power and its nature.

One important distinction which can be made between types of authority is whether it is de facto or *de jure* authority. If a person has authority by virtue of their position or role or knowledge then this is de facto authority, they are recognized as being in a position which entitles them to exercise authority. This does not mean, however, that they have been granted this power by any system or rules – *de jure* authority. The two types of authority often go together, of course, but it is not always the case, and it is important sometimes to ask about the nature of the authority being exercised. A person can also exercise different types of authority, a policeman may be a de facto authority on gardening, because of his knowledge, but this authority is not *de jure*, and he cannot compel others to apply a certain type of fertilizer. If people are using illegal fertilizer, however, he may use his *de jure* authority to arrest them. Similarly a nurse may have de facto authority, by virtue of her knowledge and experience of health care or position in a hospital, but she does not have the *de jure* authority to enforce compliance with treatment regimes.

De jure authority, where power is formally granted to people, is at the heart of political philosophy, because it does not just involve the granting of authority by the state to people, but the granting of authority by the people to the state. The questions about authority which are asked in political philosophy, therefore, concern the conditions under which authority is granted to, or claimed, by the state.

One way in which this granting can be justified is by reference to the merit of those people who make up the governing body. This idea of 'meritocracy' (government by the meritorious) can have several forms. In Plato's ideal society, governors or 'guardians' are trained from birth in philosophy and government to fit them for their task, whereas other meritocracies see birth alone as indicative of worthiness to rule – monarchists make the argument that royal birth is such an indication. Sometimes the idea of merit is tied to theological frameworks – the 'divine right of kings' is such an idea, where the royalty are seen as embodying God's law. A general feature of many meritocracy theories, however, is that those ruled have little say over the choice of their rulers or the decisions that they make – it is government for the people, not by the people.

Another way in which the granting of authority can be justified is by arguing that it is the will and choice of the people being governed. This is the basis of democratic ideas of government ('democracy' comes from the Greek *demo*, 'people' and *cracy*, 'government'). Democratic ideas of government propose that rulers are chosen or nominated by the people to act on their behalf, and presumably can be deselected if the people wish. Rulers chosen by democratic processes, as experience shows, are not necessarily good, wise or competent, and this calls into question the ability of people to choose well. The success of a democracy, therefore, depends very much on the mechanisms in place to allow people to make an informed choice. If these mechanisms are sound, however, it is possible for people to knowingly choose a government that is corrupt or foolish.

This, of course, raises the question of why people should want or need any government at all, and why they continue to abide by the decisions of their governors. One explanation for this obedience to authority was proposed by Hobbes in his discussion of the social contract. Hobbes argued that because people have an overriding desire for security in a dangerous world, they surrender their 'natural rights' to a ruling authority in exchange for social order and regulation. Hobbes suggested that rights are surrendered to a sovereign, but Locke argued that they should be surrendered to the community, or commonwealth. Locke did not advocate that individuals become secondary to the community, and the rights that they should surrender were only those which were necessary for the well-being of the community. Nor did Locke suggest that once rights were surrendered that government should proceed to do as they wished; any government should only act according to the will of the majority (see Locke, 1967).

Social contract theories seek to justify and explain why people should seek or submit to government, and their essential argument is that societies are better off with government than without. The descriptions given of the process of establishing a social contract have a quasi-historical air about them: it is almost as if these writers were chronicling a change from ungoverned to governed society. This historical interpretation is in some ways misleading, because it is not clear that these texts are actually arguing that there ever was a society without government that then decided to have it. Social contract theories do tend to infer that the choice to move towards government is a consensus decision and also that it was an explicit and rational process, whereas it is by no means certain that this is the case. Social contract theories may, however, provide some interesting explanations for societies continuing to be governed, that people recognize the value of having some regulation of society (sociologists and psychologists, however, may have other explanations).

Perhaps the most significant contribution of social contract theories, however, is the way that they emphasize the exchanges made between societies and their rulers, and therefore the conditions under which these exchanges become unsustainable. These conditions are, broadly speaking, when the state fails to fulfil its part of the bargain (in other words, it fails to provide regulation) or when it seeks to exact too much from the people (when its regulation becomes onerous or oppressive). A state which breaches its contract and exceeds its authority infringes the liberty of the people, and then becomes vulnerable – the social contract can be dissolved.

Liberty

Liberty can be seen as the other side of the coin to authority – where should authority stop? This question has occupied the minds of many political philosophers, both those whose concern has been with setting out legitimate state authority, and those who have tried to set out the principles of freedom.

Before going on to discuss ideas of freedom and liberty in political philosophy, it is useful to distinguish between two types of freedom that are postulated in much of this work. Firstly, there is 'positive freedom'; in other words, the freedom to pursue goals and choose between actions. Secondly, 'negative freedom' refers to the absence of constraints. Under this definition, people are said to be free if they are not coerced by others. There is a subtle difference between these two ideas of freedom, the difference between having opportunity or choice and not being oppressed.

Debates on liberty revolve around the possibility of conflict between the will of society in general, and the wishes of individuals in particular. Ideally, there should be no conflict, either because individuals accept the wisdom of the decisions of government, or because government simply reflects the wishes of individuals. Such consensus, however, is unlikely, as political philosophers realized, and so much of the work on liberty presupposes or hypothesizes situations where there is conflict.

J.S. Mill is one of the most famous writers to deal with this problem. Starting from the individual's point of view, he argued that there was only one justification for state interference in the liberty of the individual – the prevention of harm to others. No other reason could be supported:

> The sole end for which mankind are warranted, individually or collectively, in interfering with the liberty of action of any one of their

number is self-protection. That the only purpose for which power can be rightfully exercised over any member of a civilised community, against his will, is to prevent harm to others . . . Over himself, over his own body and mind, the individual is sovereign.

Mill's statement is important, particularly the last phrase, as it demonstrates his recognition that the state can seek to impose ideas and views on all members of society. This may be supported by the majority, but it can become oppression of minorities, suppressing all dissident voices. Mill saw the value of individualism as being the way that dissent and debate enrich and develop societies, and so suppression of opposition, apart from any other considerations, is impoverishing to cultures.

Mill distinguishes between thought and action, however, and while there is no justification for attempts to control thoughts, there is, in some circumstances, justification for controlling actions:

Acts injurious to others require a totally different treatment. Encroachment on their rights; infliction on them of any loss or damage not justified by his own rights; falsehood or duplicity in dealing with them; unfair or ungenerous use of advantage over them; even selfish abstinence from defending them against injury – these are fit objects of moral reprobation, and, in grave cases, of moral retribution and punishment.

Mill is clearly concerned with negative freedom in the way that he is at pains to limit the interference of the state or society with the freedom of the individual. In his work, however, there is also an implicit reference to positive freedom – individuals should be allowed to develop ideas and make choices in order to enrich society. This view of alternative ideas as benign (not actually harmful and potentially productive), however, seems to imply a distinction between thought and action which is not always accepted today. The idea that people can think and say what they like, as long as they do not act upon these ideas, seems to limit the notion of harm to physical injury, whereas the concept of psychological harm is now fairly commonly accepted. A racist who expresses racist views in public can be seen as inflicting psychological stress on members of other races whether or not physical action is involved.

One interesting point about Mill's work is that he makes reference to 'rights'. In debates about liberty, a common argument is that infringement of liberty violates human rights, and indeed liberty is often justified in terms of these rights. Many political philosophers refer to 'rights' in their arguments, and the term is also used in different ways in public political debates. It is therefore probably worthwhile to spend some time defining and discussing the meanings that the term can have.

Locke argued that there are some areas of a person's life which are immune from state interference, and he called these areas 'rights'. Locke's doctrine inspired the Bill of Rights in the American Constitution, which identifies areas over which the state should have no control, such as free speech. This view of rights can be seen as a negative one, in other words that there are rights to not have interference. Other writers, and certainly modern commentators have proposed a positive view of rights, in other words the right to have or do something. This positive view of rights is exemplified by debates which argue for the right to have free health care or the right to have education.

The negative notion of rights was justified by Locke as being anterior to society. In other words, that people were born with certain rights which, because they were not granted by society, could not be taken away by society. Locke's notion of rights, therefore, set the boundaries for the proper concerns of the state; when these were transgressed, the state committed an assault on the life of citizens. The positive view of rights, as the right to have or do certain things also seems to rest on the idea of natural, inborn rights which people have by virtue of the fact that they are people. Positive rights may also be justified by pragmatic, humanistic arguments, for example that if people are not helped to achieve their full potential, by giving them access to jobs, health care or education, then society as a whole will suffer because of the lost talents and unhappiness of its citizens.

One interesting point about the argument that rights are inborn rather than earned, is that it is also an argument for equality between people. Rights that people are born with are not dependent on their intelligence, wealth or social status, and so must be the same for all. This view finds expression in many legal systems in which all people are treated equally before the law, and in some health-care systems where people are treated as equal regardless of their ability to pay for health care, the likelihood of their compliance with treatment, or their potential contribution to society. If people are treated as equal in health care, then a millionaire who complies with treatment and gives money to charity receives the same care as a penniless criminal who ignores health-care advice. That this type of equality causes concern and even repugnance for some, suggests that not only are positive rights more controversial, but that the notion that all people are born equal enjoys limited acceptance with some sections of society. There is certainly an argument being implied, if not actually explicitly made, that some rights should be earned, and that some rights should be denied in certain circumstances.

Interestingly, the denial of rights is most often justified by reference to 'the common good', rather than any argument about the inequality of people. This can take the form of arguing that when there is a threat to the common good, then rights are surrendered. The argument for testing of patients for HIV without their knowledge or consent takes this form, as it is argued that the health care of all requires this information, which can only be obtained by coercion or deception. The view that some rights should be earned, however, does seem to be based on a limited acceptance of inborn rights, in other words that they are not all that extensive.

The right to infertility treatment, for example, seems to be covertly dependent on the 'suitability' of the people involved, whether this is defined as economic status or moral worthiness. In other words, whereas a woman may be seen to have an uncontested right to emergency treatment after a road accident, she may be seen to not have an equal right to infertility treatment, which is seen by some as luxury rather than a necessity. 'Luxury' health care, it seems, has to be earned, whereas 'essential' health care can be provided under the auspices of inborn rights.

Justice

The relationship between rights and equality brings us to the idea of justice. The discussion above has set out some of the arguments which form the basic principles of justice, but the practice of justice is more complicated than the simple application of these principles. 'Justice' in itself is quite an ambiguous term, but if it is taken to mean that people are to be accorded or given goods (this term meaning rights and resources rather than simply property) in a fair way, then clearly this 'fairness' involves some matching up of needs and rights. As people may have different needs, the notion of equality (especially if it is taken to mean some form of universal and uni-form treatment) obviously has to be tempered by the observation that people may have the same rights but different needs.

The problem of justice, then, is how to determine how different needs should be taken into account in the treatment of others. There are difficulties in determining the importance of needs and their extent, a difficulty demon-strated above in the reference to 'luxury' and 'essential' health care. The differences between needs cannot simply be decided by reference to their importance in maintaining life, because needs are subjectively experienced by those who have them; one person's luxury is another person's essential. Some people, for example, may habitually undergo cosmetic surgery to modify their appearance in ways which do not materially affect their quality of life, and which they recognize as being a matter of preference rather than desperate need. Someone who is severely disfigured, however, may regard the same surgery as vital to their well being. Yet again, someone who is severely disfigured may well feel that they can cope with their appearance without needing surgery.

Even if it were possible to discriminate between needs, there is still a problem in deciding what is the appropriate response. If it is accepted that people are not born equal in the sense that they are born with different talents and abilities, and in different social circumstances, then the question is raised whether justice should not be in some way concerned with correct-ing these inequalities in order that people should enjoy equal opportunities to meet their needs. This obviously suggests that resources and support should not be distributed uniformly, that, for example, a poor single parent should receive more help than an affluent couple.

Attempts to 'level the playing field', however, can meet with opposition, as proponents of ideas such as positive discrimination employment policies have found. This opposition often rests, at least in part, on the argument that it is just to reward merit. In this position, the affluent couple mentioned above are affluent because they have worked hard and deserve their affluence, whereas the single parent has not (for whatever reason) made this effort. If hard work is not to be rewarded, the argument goes, then people will not do it, and society as a whole will suffer.

Another objection is that in a state where resources are finite (that is, all states) giving extra resources to one group necessarily reduces the share available to others. Justice, then, is not simply giving to those with need, but it also involves taking away from those who are not needy. Aside from considerations of fairness, then, the exercise of justice by the state can also be regarded as an infringement on liberty: people have their resources taken away to be given to others. Where a population has some consensus about how this should be done, and the opportunity to participate in the decision-making processes involved, then the state acts according to the general will. There is still a danger, however, that people cannot participate fully in these decisions, and so may have their resources reduced against their wishes, constituting an infringement of their rights and liberty. A counterargument to this point, however, would be to say that the people most likely to be participating in state decisions are the affluent and well-educated, those who have the most resources, and so the losses that they sustain are chosen by them and likely to be minimal anyway.

One attempt to resolve these arguments has been made by Rawls, who has set out some principles under which, he argues, justice can be achieved. His first principle is that 'Each person is to have an equal right to the most extensive total system of equal basic liberties compatible with a similar system for all'. This principle sets out Rawls' view of the political foundation of justice, that the State should respect liberty or rights of the individual to the extent that is compatible with the liberty of society. In this he echoes Mill's notion of liberty as something which should be preserved unless the exercise of one person's liberty infringes another's.

Economic justice, however, is not automatic on the establishment of political justice, given that a society will inevitably have unequally distributed resources. Rawls' second principle comes in to play here:

Social and Economic inequalities are to be arranged so that they are both:

(a) to the greatest benefit of the least advantaged and

(b) attached to offices and positions open to all under conditions of fair equality of opportunity.

This principle recognizes the need to target resources so that they benefit the least advantaged (an example would be building more child health clinics in disadvantaged areas rather than affluent ones) but also that there should be an effort to ensure that opportunities for advancement should be open to all. This, in effect, asks us to put in place the conditions which would allow such equality of opportunity, such as education systems, and to avoid discriminatory practices which in some societies accord advantageous positions to limited groups in society.

Perhaps the most interesting point about Rawls' thesis is that he asks us to put ourselves in the position of the least advantaged members of society when we think about justice. Other political philosophers, Marx being the most vivid example, have taken the position of the 'underdog', but many have approached the political philosophy by looking at the concerns of the average person, or even from the perspective of the ruling classes. Making this leap of imagination, however, can be difficult to do, and some would even say that it was irrelevant. For some, the disadvantaged are not a serious consideration in politics unless they cause trouble for others, either because they have 'opted out' of society (the debate about benefits for 'New Age travellers' is an example), or because their very disadvantage calls into question their competence to function in society. For nurses and health-care workers, however, the process of viewing society from the position of those most disadvantaged is echoed in the literature on patient advocacy. A similar imaginative leap is required so that the patient's position can be understood and articulated.

Nursing and political philosophy

Professional bodies

In the introduction to this chapter we argued that nursing is largely determined by political philosophies which define concepts such as rights and justice, and underpin the authority of the state to determine health-care policies. Nursing, therefore becomes a politically determined activity in the way that it is resourced and organized. This determination exists at a professional level; in other words, how the profession of nursing is supported (or not) by the state, but also at a personal level, when nurses actually give care to patients.

There is, therefore, a strong argument that nurses should be aware of the philosophical roots of the policies that affect their practice, so that they are more able to evaluate them and think through their implications. Challenging these policies, however, is a difficult step to take. Not only is it difficult to work out appropriate methods of doing so, but there is an understandable reluctance to use patients as political weapons. What many nurses do, therefore, is to trust that their professional bodies will challenge policy on their behalf. In many ways this is a sensible thing to do (they have the experience and resources to do this), but it does not encourage political analysis of the professional body itself.

The constitution of a professional body is a political phenomena, in that the authority exercised by that body and the way that it is justified is subject to the same sorts of questions that can be asked of the state. What is the extent of the authority – are there areas which are beyond their authority, and what are the rights of the professional? How do members of the profession participate in decision-making, not only about who their leaders are, but about what they say? Is this process democratic or is it élitist? How, and in what way, are leaders accountable to professionals? Are the arguments put forward by the professional body reflective of the wishes of their members or are they in the interest of the organization itself? These questions need to be asked and answered by professions in the same way that they need to be asked of the state by its citizens. The participation of nurses in health-care policy is largely determined by professional bodies, whether these have state-granted statutory powers of jurisdiction, or whether they have derived their authority from the votes of their members, and so these matters are extremely important.

There are a number of arguments made by professional bodies to justify practices which do not seem to be democratic. One is that extensive consultation with members is expensive and time-consuming, and another is that it is impossible to share the detailed information about policy that professional bodies have access to with every member of the profession. These arguments suggest that the ability of the organization to represent its members must be taken on trust. Unconditional trust in leaders, however, can be a dangerous position to take, and so questions should then turn to the mechanisms available to ensure that this trust is justified and to detect betrayals of trust.

If nurses are satisfied with the constitution of their professional body then they have some assurance that their wishes and experiences are reflected in the political activity of that body. This political activity, however, is a cumbersome process, is not always successful and, while it is going on, nurses still have to deal with patients.

Caring for patients, as we argued in the introduction to this chapter, is not only determined by politics, but it reflects and exemplifies political philosophies. To examine this proposition further, we can look at the concepts of authority, liberty, and justice as they impinge directly on the nurse's work.

Nursing authority

Returning to the example of the child health clinic given in the introduction, one of the roles of the nurse was described as giving advice. We need, therefore to ask 'By what authority is this advice given?' If we see the basis of the authority as being the expertise and knowledge of the nurse, then this fits in with definitions of de facto authority. In other words, the nurse has extensive knowledge of child care, and is therefore acting on this authority.

Obviously, this raises questions about the extent and nature of this knowledge, and about ways of ensuring that the nurse does have it. The extent of this knowledge is often measured by formal assessment in nursing, thus we can reasonably say that if a nurse has a certain qualification, then she has a certain amount of knowledge. Without such assessment, however, we cannot be certain even of this. A student nurse who has not yet been assessed cannot be assumed to have the de facto authority that her senior colleague has.

Sometimes, however, nurses assume authority in specialized areas (or are conferred it by their patients) simply because they are a nurse *per se*, regardless of specialized knowledge. Most nurses will have experienced social occasions where complete strangers have demanded advice about their medical problems and have been disappointed when the nurse has disclaimed knowledge of that area, or declined to give advice. Sometimes they may have felt obliged to live up to expectations. This suggests that if nurses are to act and advise on the basis of their knowledge, claiming de facto authority, then they must be very clear about the extent and validity of that knowledge.

The nature of the nurse's knowledge, in other words what it is about, is also a consideration. In a child health clinic, for example, a nurse may have extensive knowledge of dietary requirements for children, but she does not necessarily know about the circumstances in which the mothers that she is advising are trying to feed their children. Her knowledge therefore, can be seen as theoretical rather than practical, and should be recognized as such. De facto authority can, therefore, be only claimed in those areas where the nurse does have knowledge.

What nurses do not have, except in limited circumstances, is *de jure* authority. In other words, they do not have the authority to compel patients to follow their instructions. They may have some delegated authority to act on behalf of the health-care organization to preserve its property and ensure that its policies are met, but they do not have general authority, given to them by any legal process, to enforce treatment regimes or to command obedience from their patients. Sometimes nurses may behave as if they do have *de jure* authority, presenting patients with no choice but to follow instructions, but this is a dangerous course to adopt.

Liberty

The limitations of nurses' authority are important to remember. This is not only because it is a usefully humbling exercise to remember these limitations, but because they also sensitize us to the issue of patient freedom. If nurses have no authority to coerce, then patients have no obligation to obey. Any compliance with nursing advice, therefore, has to be achieved through negotiation rather than the exercise of authority and patients remain free to do as they wish.

There are, however, some cases where people would want to make exceptions. These are cases where the actions of patients might cause risk to others (as in the case of someone with an infectious disease refusing to remain in quarantine) or where the patient is deemed unable to make decisions (the mentally ill or the unconscious patient would provide examples of this).

Restricting a patient's liberty where his actions are dangerous to others reflects many political philosophers who have made this point in relation to civil liberties. Applying this principle in practice, however, is fraught with difficulties, not least because of the dangers of assessing risk to others. Returning to the example of the child care clinic again, it could be argued that people have the right to bring up their children as they wish, and the state, or the nurse, cannot infringe this liberty. If, however, the nurse becomes concerned that a parent is harming a child in some way, then the liberty of the parent has to be balanced with the rights of the child to have a safe upbringing. If the risk of harm is evaluated as being great (bearing in mind the difficulties of making this assessment) then some form of coercive action might be taken – perhaps the child may be taken from the parent. This in itself, however, could be harmful to the child, and could constitute an infringement of their rights and liberty if they do not want to leave.

Not only, therefore, does a decision have to be made about whether parental action presents a risk of harm to the child, thus justifying infringement of their freedom, but an assessment has to be made of the risk that might ensue from any action taken, and whether this might infringe the liberty of the child. One argument which could be made to justify acting against the child's wishes is that the child is not capable of making the decision, because of immaturity, and so their right to remain with the parent cannot be respected. This issue of competence in decision-making as a prerequisite of having rights is also found in discussions of the liberty of people with mental illness, people with learning difficulties, and sometimes, older people. This notion of competence is inherently dangerous, suggesting as it does, that there is some standard of mental functioning which must be reached before rights can be supported. If this argument were applied wholesale, then it is quite possible that many people would find themselves without rights at all on the grounds that they were not intelligent or mature enough to make meaningful choices. Furthermore, notions of competence are essentially normative, i.e. if a person makes a decision that most people would regard as wrong, then they are, by extension, incompetent.

The position is perhaps clearer when the question of harm to others is raised. An older person who is confused and leaves the gas unlit is potentially capable of blowing up the neighbours, and this might justify some action being taken. If the person lives in an isolated house, however, and will only blow up themselves, then the question of causing harm to others is replaced by the question of whether they have the right to risk harm to themselves. People do not normally live so dangerously, and so the acceptance of risk can be seen as indicative of mental incompetence (it is unclear where this leaves rock climbers and others who pursue dangerous sports).

Virginia Henderson's definition of nursing is an interesting one in light of this debate, because it seems to imply that rights are dependent on competence. Henderson (1966) suggested that the role of the nurse was to do for the patient what they would do for themselves if they had the necessary ability and knowledge. If the patient objects to nursing intervention, then, it can be easy to attribute this to a lack of knowledge or understanding. Where patients are clearly unable to agree to interventions, for example if they are unconscious, then this might be a reasonable line of thought. Where competence is less easily assessed, however, attributing non-compliance to ignorance, and therefore justifying acting against the patient's expressed wishes is a dubious course of action.

Acting in areas which the patient regards as their area of jurisdiction is an infringement of negative rights (see above). It is, however, also possible to infringe positive rights. For example, many health-promotion strategies are based on the naive assumption that if you tell people what is good for them, then they will do it. The corollary of this argument is that if they do not comply with advice, then they are either ignorant or wilful. Arguing wilful non-compliance paves the way for withdrawing health care – a sanction which infringes positive rights to health care although it preserves the negative right of protection against undue intrusion.

Justice in nursing

Another argument for withdrawing health care from non-compliant patients is that it is a waste of resources. If resources are finite, then, the argument goes, they must be targeted to areas where they are most effective. This is a different argument to that made by some political philosophers about justice, particularly Rawls (1972), an argument based on need rather than effectiveness. If justice consists of giving to those in greatest need, then resources might be expended with little success, but this is not a central consideration of some arguments about justice. Others, however, would argue for a merit-based distribution of resources. In this argument, effectiveness becomes evidence that the right decision was made.

Building child care clinics in deprived areas fulfils Rawls' principles of justice in that it arranges inequalities to the greatest benefit of those least advantaged. Building child care clinics in better-off neighbourhoods, where parents are more able and willing to follow advice, fulfils merit-based notions of justice. The people in the better-off areas deserve such provision as a reward for their hard work and sense of responsibility.

Building clinics is an obvious distribution of resources, but there are other resources which are distributed in health care. In the child health clinic described in the introduction to this chapter, the resources in question are the nurse's time and energy, but the arguments about justice prevail whatever the type of resource. In the example we gave, the nurse was faced with a dilemma about how she should spend her time. Should she give more to the parent with problems (and therefore less to the others)? Giving more time to the parents with problems meets Rawls' requirements for justice as it is to the benefit of the parent who is least advantaged. The other parents do not need as much time, and it is also possible that time spent with the disadvantaged parent will be more effective in terms of improving quality of life for that person. The point could be made, however, that the other parents are deprived of time with the nurse. This point seems in part to be based on the idea that justice means giving the same to everyone, and as such does not take into account differing needs. Allotting a strict ten minutes for every parent at the clinic could mean that some parents do not have the opportunity to discuss their problems, while others are forced to make small-talk until their time is up. This type of nonsensical situation can also be found in other areas of nursing, where there is the concern to treat everyone the same, in the interests of fairness. Nurses, therefore, become paranoid about accusations of favouritism and preferential treatment if they deviate from the norm. Patients are restricted to the same number of visitors at their bedside, eat at the same time as others, have the same number of baths, and are generally treated as if they were identical, in the interests of fairness.

This view of justice not only fails to address the question of different needs among patients, but it also does not fit with ideas of individualized care which are so prevalent in the nursing literature. Individualized care has been advocated precisely because it is a way of differentiating between patients; it rests on the observation that different patients have different needs. What the literature has failed to do, however, is discuss how different needs can be met within a community of patients; how the needs of one patient can be juggled with the needs of others. If individualized nursing care is to be the way that nursing develops these questions must be debated, and reference to the wider philosophical debates on justice can only help this debate.

Conclusion

Ideas about politics, the best way to run a state, what the ideas of freedom and justice mean, are of immediate relevance to nursing. They not only determine the large-scale organization of health care, but also affect the immediate decisions that nurses make on the point of delivering care. Whether nurses work in a health-care system which allocates health care on the basis of ability to pay, or which sees health care as a right, they are working in a politically directed system.

Ideas and debates in political philosophy, however, can also help to inform many current debates about nursing practice and theory. The link between ideas of justice and concepts of individualized care has been referred to, but there are many other links which it is possible to make. Humanistic psychology, for example, which stresses the facilitation of personal development, can be linked to ideas about equality of opportunity, and ideas about liberty can be helpful in putting nursing intervention in context.

Political ideas are not, of course, the sole determinant of nursing practice, but their importance is undeniable. Some would argue that politics is simply about what happens in the political world and that nursing practice takes place in a different, personal arena. Feminist theorists have argued, however, that the personal is political, and in many ways this chapter has tried to make these links clearer. The common concerns of nurses and political philosophers are closer than many would think (or wish!).

References

Hegel, G.W.F. 1956: *Lectures on the philosophy of history.* New York: Dover.
Henderson, V. 1966: *The nature of nursing.* New York: Macmillan.
Hobbes, T. 1972: *Leviathan.* London: Collins.
Huxley, A. 1932: *Brave New World.* London: Chatto and Windus.
Locke, J. 1967: *Two treatises of government.* Cambridge: Cambridge University Press.
Mill, J.S. 1982: *On liberty.* Harmondsworth: Penguin.
Orwell, G. 1962: *1984.* London: Secker and Warburg.
Rawls, J. 1972: *A theory of justice.* Oxford: Oxford University Press.
Rousseau, J.J. 1968: *The social contract.* London: Penguin.

Further reading

Arendt, H. 1973: *On revolution.* Harmondsworth: Penguin.
Aristotle, 1981: *Politics.* Harmondsworth: Penguin.
Nozick, R. 1975: *Anarchy, state and Utopia.* Oxford: Blackwell.
Machievelli, N. 1992: *The prince.* London: David Campbell.
More, T. 1964: *Utopia.* Newhaven, CT: Yale University Press.
Plato 1955: *The republic.* Harmondsworth: Penguin.
Plamenatz, J.P. 1963: *Man and society.* London: Longman.
Quinton, A. (ed.) 1967: *Political philosophy.* Oxford: Oxford University Press.
Sabine, G.H. 1963: *History of political theory.* London: Harrap.
Soper, K. 1990: *Troubled pleasures: writings on politics, gender and hedonism.* Oxford: Blackwell.
Wollstonecraft, M. 1975: *A vindication of the rights of women.* Harmondsworth: Penguin.

Philosophy of language

8

Introduction

For some people, the philosophy of language epitomises what is worst about philosophy. The idea that it is profitable to discuss definitions and terms, rather than actions and events, suggests an 'ivory tower' mentality at its extreme. In the end, is philosophy not just about words? – just playing around with words, mere 'semantics', unconnected with the wards and worlds of nursing practice? Certainly there is a sense in which philosophy is about words. But this is just why philosophy does matter to practical matters. For it is in words that we say what we mean; it is in words that we argue, persuade and protest. And it is with words that we can care, nurture and heal. Though it is also with words that we can humiliate, offend and fob off.

A brief excursion into nursing history shows that nursing, a practical discipline, has been very much concerned with words and terms – and with good reason. For example, some readers may remember nursing at a time when patients were referred to only by their bed number or by their diagnosis, and if names were used to avoid confusion between patients, this was the only acknowledgement of their individuality. Starting a shift, a nurse would be given a report which baldly listed names, ages and diagnoses, with a brief summary of progress or decline. The use of language in this way both reinforced and expressed a view of the patient as a series of tasks, distinguishable from others only by diagnosis or bed number, and there was some disquiet at this dehumanizing approach. As nursing moved towards a view of patients as unique individuals, the stark language of the ward report became inadequate for the new approach, and so the language began to change. Patients were not referred to as 'the hernia in bed twelve' but as 'Mr Smith, who has a hernia'. The change, of course, was not immediate or absolute, but those who had not changed became remarkable for their outdated approach.

For those who dispute the importance of words, these changes are merely cosmetic and of no real significance for practice. Referring to someone as 'a hernia', however, immediately conveys a different set of concerns and attitudes to referring to someone as a *person* who has a hernia. In the former, the impression is one of a mechanistic focus on physical condition, whereas the latter conveys respect or at least acknowledgement of the person, with their particular identity and personality, who has the condition. If the distraught relatives hear the nurse telling her colleague that 'The appendectomy in bed fourteen is dead', it will be no good protesting that these are only words. Words carry meaning. Additionally this meaning is not restricted to the listener; it is difficult to conceive of a nurse using a particular form of language, whether depersonalized or humanized, without conveying something to her- or himself.

Understanding how words have meaning and how it is that with words, we can mean anything at all, has been a central task for an important subdepartment of philosophy – the philosophy of language. This branch of philosophy has only fairly recently grown in importance, although language has, of course, been the essential medium of philosophical debate. It was, however, 'taken for granted', as a relatively unproblematic facet of life. More recently, however, language has been paid much attention in modern analytical philosophy. It is as if language was transparent, very much as a pane of glass in a window is – we concentrate on the view beyond. Now, however, language has lost its transparency – we are examining the pane of glass itself.

Philosophical ideas about language have taken two broad forms. In the first language is treated as a set of symbols which 'map onto' the world, and as such is amenable to the laws of logic, and should be analysed in this way. Language problems here are conceived of as problems of accuracy and clarity, and the solution to these problems is to develop a language which is crystal clear in its meaning. This traditional way of thinking about language can be traced back to the ancient Greeks, whose primary concerns were with metaphysical inquiries about the nature of reality, asking questions such as: Are there numbers? Does The Good exist? Are values unchangeable? This quest for the nature of reality led to some problems. Because we often assume that the world as depicted by science of the time tells us what is real, we trust the scientist to deliver the data (psychology or physics or biology) and then we see what implications these have. Then we may get dissatisfied with the ability of language to represent this reality. We talk about linguistic inadequacy or more radically start to design a purified language that be perfectly suited to the nature of reality – logical, pure, crystalline in its simplicity. Von Leibniz (1973) dreamed of a universal characteristic, Frege (1979) made us see what it might be like and it was pursued by the early Wittgenstein (1961).

The second form of analysis looks at the way that language is used to make sense of the world. There is no assumption of direct correlation between words and the world; indeed, this type of relationship is strongly challenged. Many of the debates in nursing about language seem to echo the former approach, which is why such debates run into the problems inherent in this view of language. In this chapter we show why understanding the nature and use of language is important to resolving some of the disputes that characterize many debates about the character of nursing.

The problem with language

A characteristic problem in discussions about the nature of nursing is that there is disagreement, not just about what we should do, but about the very terms used in the discussion. This can lead to the type of debate which is often justifiably dismissed as wrangling about words. The debates, however, can often become bogged down by two particular problems, and it is by understanding the nature of these problems that we may be able to find some way around them. The first is the problem of trying to find precise and unambiguous definitions, and the second is the problem of avoiding definitions which can be seen as derogatory – the 'political correctness' ('PC' as it is often known) problem. For nurses, the problem is to be precise about what terms mean, so that the words used can be universally understood, but to avoid the use of terms which stereotype patients, and take away the individuality that they wish to recognize and make fundamental to care.

Disputes over definitions

For some people, we can only talk sensibly about a particular topic in nursing if we can clearly define all the terms that we use. For example, some professional debates about appropriate care for the 'elderly' quickly become bogged down in two kinds of dispute. The first kind of dispute concerns the meaning of the term 'elderly'. What exactly do we mean by this term? Different people have offered different definitions. For some, the term refers simply to people of a particular age. This looks straightforward so long as we put off answering the obvious question of what age we have in mind. Sixty? Sixty-five? Eighty-five? For others, the term is to be defined in terms of certain abilities or, perhaps more likely, the loss of certain abilities. For yet others, it seems best, since the term is to be used in a nursing context, to give it a meaning in terms of health status. And for others, it is economic status that counts. The elderly are those who are no longer economically active.

What creates the dispute over this term is that there will always be individuals who do not fall in the specified category. And so the definitions seem inadequate. If we cannot really define exactly what we mean by the 'elderly', how can we hope to discuss and understand the role of the nurse in relation to them? One response to some problems of definition is to argue that if we cannot agree a water-tight, all-purpose definition, then it is no good talking about the matter at all. If we cannot agree what we mean by the 'elderly', what is the point in discussing it? This sort of definitional dispute is based partly on the idea of language 'mapping onto' the world. If we cannot find a word to map onto a phenomenon, to represent it exactly, then either our language is inadequate, or the phenomenon does not exist.

The PC problem

Another dispute is, where we have been able to define the terms, whether these terms are pejorative. 'Old people', 'geriatric', 'elderly people', 'senior citizens', 'OAPs' and 'Grey Panthers' are all terms that have been used to describe older people, but they differ very much in the images that they convey. 'Geriatric' has become pejorative, 'senior citizens' is more respectful and 'grey panthers' is positively racy. A similar dispute for nurses and other health-care workers is whether the people that they care for should be called 'patients', 'clients' or 'customers', a debate which reflects not only changes in professional attitudes but also political changes. We can call people customers if we like but that in itself does not guarantee that they will want to buy anything, although it does emphasize a contractual aspect of health care. Some would argue that using the term 'customer' makes us more likely to value people, conjuring up as it does someone who has opinions, choices and preferences about the care which is bought. Seeing people as customers who might (theoretically at least) go elsewhere if they are not satisfied emphasizes the idea that health care is for the recipients rather than the providers of services.

Opponents of the 'customer' terminology argue that this reduces the relationship between nurses and the people that they care for to a commercial transaction, and this fails to capture the moral and personal dimensions of nursing work. Being a customer of health care is not the same as buying baked beans in a supermarket, and the relationship with the nurse is not the same as the relationship with the cashier. Talking about Mrs Jones as a 'patient' stresses the specific, health-care-related nature of the relationship between her and the nurse (and that is why we have tended to use it in this book). If, however, this is only the language we use, we reduce Mrs Jones to a 'bit of' herself – it ignores the other dimensions of Mrs Jones. Moreover, the 'bit of' Mrs Jones that we highlight when calling her a patient does not have rights in the same way that a customer does.

This type of language problem owes something to the idea that language should map perfectly onto what it describes, where the problem is seen as being with the exact characteristics of people receiving care and their matching with the exact terms which precisely denote these characteristics. At the same time, however, there is another concern, not with the accuracy of our words, but with the use to which we put them. By calling someone a 'customer' of health care, some would argue that we empower them, while others would argue that we demean them. Language, then, is not just a matter of matching objects with words, but it carries a moral and political dimension in the way that we use it.

Philosophical reactions

The problems that nurses experience in using language are not, of course, unique to nursing – they arise in many areas of life. Philosophy has responded to and examined these dilemmas, and the arguments that have developed are of great use to those trying to find their way around these impasses.

The definitional problem

The philosophical view underlying this kind of problem is this: every meaningful term can be exhaustively defined in terms of a set of conditions which govern its application. To describe the kind of definition that people have in mind here, logicians use a distinction between necessary and sufficient conditions. Something is a *necessary condition*, say of being elderly, if no one can be said to be elderly unless this is true of them. So, it is a necessary condition of being elderly that one is at least alive! But obviously not all living people are elderly. Something is a *sufficient condition*, say of being elderly, if, given that this is true of someone, then they must be elderly. So, it is a sufficient condition of being elderly if one is, say, 101 years old. But this may not be all there is to being elderly.

Very often disputes about terminology arise because what one person offers as a necessary condition, another interprets as a sufficient condition and vice versa. So, someone claims that not being able to look after oneself is a necessary condition of being elderly. Another replies, irrelevantly, that this cannot be true because many young people are not able to look after themselves. Again, someone claims that if someone is suffering medical condition X, then they must be elderly. The other replies, irrelevantly, that there is more than that to being elderly. Should we only use terms where we can supply a full set of necessary and sufficient conditions? The temptation to think so is very strong. After all, we may think, unless we can always say if someone is elderly or not, we do not know what we mean by this term. Unless all cases of being 'elderly' have something in common, how can we talk about the elderly as a group?

It may be thought that supplying these cast-iron definitions is precisely the kind of job that philosophers should be doing. One conclusion that has emerged from the philosophy of language, however, is that it is, at least sometimes, a mistake to think that such definitions are always necessary, or that we only understand what we mean if we are in possession of such a definition. In short, the meaning of a word need not consist of a set of necessary and sufficient conditions for its correct application.

First of all, it must be pointed out that most of us, most of the time, find it pretty difficult to supply such definitions even for terms which we do not think are especially problematic. We are all pretty familiar with the word 'cat'. We can pick out cats, even cats with very different physical appearances, distinguish them from dogs and so on. But how many of us can supply anything like a set of necessary and sufficient conditions for something's being a cat? If we reflect on this, we may be inclined to think that we must somehow or other know this definition for, otherwise, how could we even use the word? Perhaps we know the meaning of the word 'cat' unconsciously. One trouble with this view is that there is no evidence that supports it. A worse problem is that it is hard to know what use an unconscious grasp of the meaning would be. Worst of all, it is clear that these sets of necessary and sufficient conditions would have themselves to be in the medium of words, and therefore subject to the same sort of problem. We seem now to be in a real mess.

The philosopher Ludwig Wittgenstein claimed that this whole way of thinking about the meaning of words was a deep-seated and systematic error. He asks us to consider the example of the word 'game' (Wittgenstein, 1967).

> Consider for example the proceedings that we call 'games'. I mean board-games, card-games, ball-games, Olympic games, and so on. What is common to them all? – Don't say: 'There must be something common, or they would not be called "games"' – but look and see whether there is anything common to all. For if you look at them you will not see something that is common to all, but similarities, relationships, and a whole series of them at that. To repeat: do not think, but look! Look for example at board-games, with their multifarious relationships. Now pass to card-games; here you find many correspondences with the first group, but many common features drop out, and others appear. When we pass next to ball-games, much that is common is retained, but much is lost. Are they are all 'amusing'? Compare chess with noughts and crosses. Or is there always winning and losing, or competition between players? Think of patience. In ball-games there is winning and losing; but when a child throws his ball at the wall and catches it again, this feature has disappeared. Look at the parts played by skill and luck; and at the difference between skill in chess and skill in tennis. Think now of games like ring-a-ring-a-roses; here is the element of amusement, but how many other characteristic features have disappeared! And we can go though the many, many other groups of games in the same way; can see how similarities crop up and disappear.
>
> And the result of this examination is: we see a complicated network of similarities overlapping and criss-crossing sometimes similarities in the large and sometimes similarities in the small.

Wittgenstein's portrayal of language suggests that the way we use words is not with regard to their ability to 'map onto' the world in any exact way. Rather, he suggests that we use a notion of 'family resemblance'. In much the same way as a family of people can have some resemblance which enables us to recognize them as members of the same family without them all necessarily having the same shape of nose or colour of hair, we can recognize family resemblance between phenomena, and we are quite happy to use language this way. Moreover, other people generally understand us when we do so.

The idea of family resemblance was demonstrated by Wittgenstein by reference to the word 'game'. When we think about it carefully, we can see that all of the things we call games have no one defining characteristic. Not all games are fun, not all games are entertainment. Not all games are physical, not all involve spectators, not all involve rules. Every time we think of a possible defining characteristic, we immediately think of an exception, yet we still continue to use the word without too much trouble.

Wittgenstein also extended this idea of games to language in general, when he talked of different kinds of language games. In other words, language can be used to do different things in different contexts, for example in discussing science or in debating religious ideas. Rather than all of these uses of language being amenable to the same sort of logical analysis, they all have their different forms of discourse. Telling a joke, for example, is not subject to analysis based on its accuracy or precision, and if a joke teller is met with a response which suggests that the audience is trying to do this, then it is reasonable to conclude that the audience has 'no sense of humour'. A joke is not a statement of empirical fact, and most of us recognize this – different rules apply.

Wittgenstein's idea was that the way we play language games is generally rule-governed, i.e. we know what is appropriate, how words are to be taken and what are the limits of the game. This is not to say that he thought that rules were inflexible or could be taken for granted; indeed, he observed that rule systems always had gaps in them – rules cannot provide for all eventualities. Furthermore, rules are subject to different interpretations, and these interpretations only converge through participation in shared social practices: going along together in the same way. Obeying rules, however, is a social practice, and one that is learned and complied with. The language game of having a consultation with a doctor, for example, has been the subject of much social research, some of which has described instances where patients break rules (for example, answering in full when the doctor asks how they are) and how they are 'taught' to comply (the doctor completely ignores them).

Wittgenstein's emphasis on the social nature of language also led him to argue that there is no such thing as a 'private language'; in other words, we do not use words to name inner sensations that no-one else could understand. This is an important argument, as there is a tradition in philosophy that regards knowledge as developing 'from the inside out', i.e. we start with inner private sensations and then construct public language. Wittgenstein argued that this is not how language works – we can only name inner sensations because there is already a public language. Furthermore, he argued that a private language is impossible because we would never know if we were right in our naming. If for example, I had an inner sensation and called it 'X' then the next time I had a sensation, I would not be able to decide whether it should be named X or Y without some sort of external criteria.

Wittgenstein's description of how language is used can be taken to suggest a non-problematic, consensual view, and indeed one of his concerns was to describe how language works. The problems of language that we have discussed in this chapter, however, suggest that language is sometimes very problematic indeed. The problems arise, Wittgenstein suggests, not because there is something wrong with language, because we have failed to pay attention to the way that it is being used, and the language game to which it belongs. In these circumstances, Wittgenstein argued 'language goes on holiday'.

Wittgenstein's description of language games was developed in his later philosophy, most particularly in his 'Philosophical Investigations', which was published after his death. His later ideas contrasted with his earlier work, the Tractatus Logico-philosophicus, in which he had argued for a more precise and exact understanding of language and its limits, and it is worth mentioning it here in order to see how he had changed. The Tractatus, which begins with the impressive and unequivocal statement that 'The world is everything that is the case', argued that the world is made of 'Facts' or states of affairs. A fact might be that there is a chair in this room. The business of language is to picture facts. Logical analysis of the language used in propositions can reveal the structure of the facts that make up the world. Propositions which do not picture facts, for example expressions of religious belief, are, strictly speaking meaningless.

The Tractatus was received with great enthusiasm by a group of philosophers known as the logical positivists, who lived mainly in Vienna in the 1920s. They developed Wittgenstein's idea of elementary propositions in several ways, one of which was to equate elementary propositions with empirical experiences. This perhaps reflected the academic background of many members, who were scientists rather than philosophers, but the concern with empirical experiences was also a reaction to some of the very abstract metaphysical debate which was taking place in philosophy at the time.

Wittgenstein, however, moved on from the Tractatus, and in his later work challenged the centrality of the logical analysis of language and the limits that he had identified for it. He began to reflect that everyone (even philosophers) manages to get by using language in ways that are not amenable to logical scrutiny and about things which are not facts. The question that then became prominent was, 'How can this be?' When Wittgenstein began to consider how language is used, rather than how it should be used, he came to a very different understanding of it, which addressed its social and interactive aspects. His later work, the Philosophical Investigations, demonstrates this change and his ideas about language games, which we outlined above, are very different from the Tractatus.

As a demonstration of the practical use of Wittgenstein's later ideas, we can look at his war work. During World War II, he joined a research team, which was for some time based in Newcastle upon Tyne (Monk, 1990). The team were looking at the treatment of shock which occurs as the result of traumatic injury and can lead to cardiovascular collapse. Wittgenstein's official role in this team was as a technician, but his contribution was also important in shaping the way in which the team thought about shock. The problem that the team had was that there seemed to be no clear way of defining shock, as much of the data from World War I was incomplete, inaccurate or contradictory. Some clinicians used symptoms such as pallor and sweating to identify the condition, while others used high red blood cell counts. In discussions with Reeve and Grant, the doctors leading the team, Wittgenstein was enthusiastic about abandoning the term – even suggesting that in the final report the term should be printed upside down to indicate its uselessness. In short, he believed, as did the rest of the team, that it is useless to look for a precise definition of shock, and it is only possible to describe the conditions of people who have experienced major trauma. Cases of shock have a family resemblance, and it is a mistake to think that there is an 'essence' of shock which can be used to distinguish cases. It is not that sort of language game.

The PC problem – the philosophical response

One distinction from the philosophy of language that can prove useful in this context is that between what we do in speaking and what effect our speaking produces. In other words, we can think of language as a set of 'speech acts' which do things, rather than some neutral medium through which we simply report or convey acts.

Let us first look at the idea that profound political change in society can be produced by conscious manipulation of the language of that society. Note the term 'conscious', for we are not concerned here with those changes in vocabulary which accompany political changes. The terms 'yuppies', 'dinkies', 'woopies' and so on, may now sustain, nourish and generate new instances of the groups they describe but, originally, they were responses to the factionalization of our society, not planned causes of that process. The idea of consciously planned linguistic change for political ends is, of course, a very old idea indeed. Empire builders have always known that a vital tool in turning an independent culture into one dependent upon the invader is the destruction of the home language. The English have been particularly adept at this. But deliberately setting out to destroy a language with the idea of replacing it with a existing one is different both from setting out to create a new one from scratch and from the conscious manipulation of the existing, dominant, language.

Historically, this latter strategy is characteristic not of imperialism but of revolution. And indeed, perhaps the most radical attempt to self-consciously manipulate a language for political ends was that practised by the theorists of the French Revolution. Certainly some of the changes proposed and adopted were relatively trivial – changes in the names of clothes and food dishes – one, somewhat bizarre, relic of these changes is Lobster Thermidore. But the revolution also had ambitions concerning the vocabulary governing more important matters. Indeed it is difficult to think of areas of more profound metaphysical importance than those on which the radicals of the revolution concentrated their efforts, i.e. time, space and human relations. There were changes in the structure and vocabulary of the seasons, the calendar and the time of day. Pre-revolutionary systems of measuring distance, volume and size were replaced with a new 'metric' and even the structure of relations between the new citizens was to be newly created by

abandoning the formal pronoun 'vous'. Henceforth, all citizens are as broth-
ers and sisters in a new time and a new space. It may be that one legacy of
this has been those official French committees deciding whether or not 'Le
Weekend' is be allowed into the culture. A practice which, no doubt because
we have not been on the receiving end of linguistic imperialism for some
time, the English find ever so faintly embarrassing. But there have been other
less amusing legacies too. When we are struck by the chill horror of Cam-
bodia's Day Zero we should perhaps remember that Pol Pot was drawing
upon an established, essentially liberal, progressive, European tradition.

Now, there are many questions we can ask about the idea of deliberately
conceived changes in language for political ends. But one of the difficulties is
working out just what in any particular case is supposed to be happening.
Here are some of the possibilities, each illustrated by the example of the
decree made during the French Revolution, that the formal term 'vous'
should not be used, and instead citizens should refer to each other by the
more egalitarian term 'tu':

- The linguistic change commemorates a political change. So, abandoning
'vous' as a pronoun might be analogous to renaming a square 'Place de la
Revolution'.
- The linguistic change acts as an mnemonic for political change. So,
abandoning 'vous' might simply serve as a reminder to citizens that an
important change has taken place. Every time they talk to someone they
will be consciously reminded of their new status as citizens.
- The linguistic change acts as an symbol or metaphor for political change.
Like the mnemonic but more subtle, subliminal even, in its effects.
- The linguistic change assists in facilitating political change by removing
existing barriers to change. This might be because the form 'vous' originally commemorated, or reminded citizens, or symbolized or acted as
metaphor for the old order and harking back to the past impedes
change. But this is a kind of half-way house on our progress. For the
form 'vous' may be a barrier not because it now reminds citizens of the
old order but just because it actively sustained the old order in one of a
number of ways: the same ways as those in which the abandonment of the
term may be intended to consolidate the new order.
- The linguistic change makes possible a political change which speakers of
the language may independently desire. How, as a matter of fact, might
linguistic change make political change possible? Perhaps by what philosophers of language call a 'Gricean reflexive mechanism'. The new citizens want to treat and be treated by their citizens as equals. Now if,
simply as a matter of fact, everyone only uses 'tu', this will not mean
that everyone is treated by, and as, equals. Surely, just to use the words is
not enough? But, if everyone knows that everyone has decided to use 'tu'
just in order to bring it about that everyone is treated by, and as, equals,
then simply by using only 'tu', one indicates one's choice that one would
indeed treat the other as an equal. Think of it the other way around. As
Lenny Bruce pointed out, the words 'nigger', 'spick' and 'pommy' are not

intrinsically offensive or insulting words. Possibly they may all originally have been neutrally descriptive. But as a matter of fact, they have been the words used by those intending to offend members of the respective groups. Given this and given, crucially, that everyone knows that everyone is acquainted with this fact, then it is impossible to think that one might not run the risk of being thought to be choosing to be insulting or offensive by using such words. But if so, then, knowing this, to deliberately choose to use such a word is, *ipso facto*, to choose to insult or offend a member of one of those groups. In this way then, the linguistic change makes possible a political change which speakers of the language may independently desire and later choose.

- The linguistic change makes possible a political change which speakers of the language may desire only when the linguistic change has taken effect. The citizens can imagine nothing other than the old class system. Because of this, the 'tu/vous' distinction seems perfectly natural. But, when they are eventually cajoled or coerced into using only 'tu', they come to see that the old 'tu/vous' distinction was in fact very artificial. They then see that the social distinctions it marked were also entirely artificial. They are now able to imagine a new way of life which they may or may not come to prefer.

All of these might be true descriptions of the relation between linguistic and political change. It is by no means an exhaustive list of possibilities. But at least those described are all different from that envisaged by Orwell, in his novel *1984*. In this book, Orwell imagined a state which deliberately enforced changes in language, and called this Newspeak. Newspeak differs from the descriptions suggested above in these two crucial respects: firstly the linguistic change does not make possible but actually brings about the political change, and secondly the political change is not one which may be desired independently of the linguistic change. Nor is it one which may be desired only and independently after the linguistic change. Rather, the political change is one which can, and must, be desired after the linguistic change.

Another interesting approach to the relationship between the words that we use and the feelings or attitudes that they express is formulated in the Sapir–Whorfian hypothesis. These American linguists have proposed that the concepts we use are determined by the language that we use, and therefore our world view differs according to the language that we use. Whorf's (1956) research into the language of the Hopi Indians had concluded that their language lacks tenses, and they therefore do not use concepts such as time in the way that other language speakers use them. This hypothesis is a tempting one – it has often been observed, for example, that the British use French words such as 'chic' or 'sang-froid' to talk about styles of dress or social poise. The conclusion that the British are totally devoid of dress sense or social graces, however, requires empirical observation of the clothes that are worn and the manners they display, rather than the language they use. It may well be argued that the British culture has not produced equivalent words because the British have not, historically, been concerned with these things, but there is also other evidence that fashion and manners have been very much at the centre of British life. The Sapir–Whorfian hypothesis seems, therefore, to simplify the relationship between language and thought in a seductive, but ultimately unhelpful way.

Another, more widely known, approach to looking at language comes form the post-modernists, particularly from the method of textual analysis called 'deconstruction'. Post-modernism, as the name implies, is a reaction to modernism, the idea that civilization is progressing through rationality and science. The problems with this view, which began with the Enlightenment ideas of science, have been observed by many writers and philosophers, but also by scientists, architects and musicians, to name but a few disciplines. The modernist view incorporates meta-narratives about society, for example Marxism which sees society as largely about economic forces, or Freudian theory which sees it as governed by the unconscious, or feminist theory which sees it as the structured oppression of women. These are seen as universal structures which can be 'decoded' to tell us what is going on in the world. Alongside these meta-narratives are ideas of absolutes or essences that, for example, there are such things as a classic play, unquestionable moral rules, eternal family structures, or innate gender differences which endure throughout time, and somehow stand outside history and culture.

The post-modernist objections to this are that the modernist view takes too much for granted: that Shakespeare is a great playwright, that immunization is a good thing, that the free market is the only way to run businesses. All of these things are not absolute truths, but are part of the cultural and social context in which they are placed. Immunization, for example, was initially seen as an unnatural thing to do, then became a triumph of medicine, and in the future may become a discredited practice. What post-modernists argue is that modernism itself is simply a story or narrative that is currently privileged (given more weight and importance) in our culture, but it is not the only possible story, and that we should look for others.

Post-modernism offers another critique of the view that language 'maps onto' objects in the way that it challenges the notion of objects. Rather than objects being taken for granted as universal and unproblematic, the post-modernist argument asserts that there are many different perspectives and views to take, and distinguishing between them cannot involve straightforward appeals to rationality. In other words, there is no one right way, but a multiplicity of ways of seeing the world, of talking about it and telling stories about it.

Revealing these ways involves a process of deconstruction, of taking language and examining it closely, and this is worth doing because in this way language can be challenged and examined for the values it exhibits. In particular, language and texts can be examined according to the cultural and historical context of which they are a part. A historical text, for example, is not a straightforward reporting of facts and figures, because the writing of the text involves a process of selection, and this selection is determined by the cultural context in which the text is written. Historical accounts of the British Empire, for example, might have been written in Victorian times as exciting exploits of brave men pushing back the frontiers of civilization. A more recent text could well focus on the ill-treatment of native people and the exploitation of natural resources. This is not to say that the authors of these respective books were lying, or even consciously manipulating facts – it is simply that their work is part of the cultural milieu in which it is written, and therefore cannot be separated from it. In this sense, the authors of these texts are less 'in control' than presumed. They have to use a language which is intelligible to others and to themselves, and they must construct a text accordingly which contains elements which are as much a creation of the culture in which they live as of them as individuals.

A feminist, who had overcome her objections to post-modernist anti-structuralism, might deconstruct language to reveal how it takes the masculine gender to represent women too, for example in the use of the term 'mankind' to represent everyone. Foucault (1976), in his examination of the history of medicine, showed how the modernist 'rational' progress of medicine could also be seen as a process of colonization. As and because medicine gained in prestige, doctors began to assume an expertise in areas of life which had not been thought of as medical at all. Current debates about crime illustrate this point – what has been a simple matter of morality, with criminals committing crimes because of their 'badness', is now part of a medical debate about hormones, nutrition and genes. The deconstruction of texts and language prevents us from taking for granted that they represent 'the world in itself', and allow us to trace the historical development of a concept and how it has been constructed.

The tool of deconstruction, however, is an extremely complicated one to use, and attracts much dissent, even among post-modernists. At one extreme post-modernism can be criticized for trying to show what a text or a speech 'really means', in contradiction to the idea of multiple meaning. On the other hand, if a pluralistic view is adopted, it can be criticized for dismissing values. If post-modernism starts to looks as if it is suggesting that there are only words or perspectives, it can be criticized for dismissing the structures and inequalities of the material world (the point at which the feminist might have problems). However, if having deconstructed language it looks as if it is trying to point to how the material world is, it begins to look as if it is returning to a simple mapping notion of language.

Perhaps the value of post-modernism lies in the general point that it makes about language, that it is not a neutral vehicle for the conveying of ideas and facts, but it can shape and direct our responses in ways that we would do well to think about. This idea of reflexivity, of analysing text and language and our responses to it, exhorts us to a discipline of reading and listening that prevents us from taking things for granted. The notion of a multiplicity of ways of telling stories and thinking about things is also a useful thought to have. The problem, however, is what we do next.

This can be illustrated by looking at the debates in post-modernist psychotherapy. One view of psychotherapy is that it is about finding out what people's problems are, and then suggesting solutions. In post-modernist therapy, however, there is an acceptance that there are different stories possible. An adolescent taking drugs might be simply immoral, crying out for help, lacking in confidence, biologically vulnerable to addiction, or simply full of enthusiasm for new experiences according to different stories. A post-modernist therapist would explore all of these narratives, taking care not to privilege one over the other, particularly their own. Once these stories have been told, however, the therapist has a problem about what to do next, given that the adolescent's family have come to therapy with what they see as a problem, and want some answers. One response is to argue that the therapist's job is to find the story which best allows change, or which is most comfortable to live with, but this notion of choosing the 'best' story contradicts many of the post-modernist exhortations to celebrate difference and diversity, and to value all narratives equally. To let the matter rest after the telling of the stories, however, does not seem to be enough to either alleviate the family's distress, stop the drug-taking or justify the therapist's salary. While post-modernism has been useful in opening up the possibilities of narrative it cannot, and would not claim to tell us what to do next.

Conclusion

These philosophical debates can be linked back to the problems that nurses experience when debating language. To return to the problem of finding words to talk about older people, the problem can be summarized thus: if we say the 'elderly' cannot be defined, how can we sensibly talk about them? On the other hand, if we can define them, do we run the risk of stereotyping them? The feeling is that we can only talk about them as a group if we understand what makes them members of that group – if we pigeon-hole them. But we should not put real individual people in pigeon-holes.

What we need, therefore, is to think of language use rather than language accuracy, and to use the notion of family resemblance, rather than search for exact characteristics which will make our use of words automatic and unquestionable. We can then talk of 'the elderly' as a term which does not convey universally shared characteristics in the group that it refers to, but as a term which covers a range of different characteristics, lifestyles and health problems, none of which being found in all members of the group. In this way, the term becomes a useful way of thinking about needs and policies, rather than a pigeon-hole to put people in.

This does not mean that language is unimportant, as we also need to recognize that the language we use is not something separate from what we are doing in using it. The examples of disputes over PC terms is an example of this recognition, in that the way language is used can be pejorative, because language can become offensive. As nurses we need to be careful and thoughtful about our language precisely because we 'do things' with our words – we comfort, admonish, demean and support with what we say. Furthermore, we need to be aware of these complexities when we listen to those that we care for; their language 'does things' too. The patient who politely agrees to comply with treatment and then does not is perhaps playing a different language game to us. If we are playing the game of 'giving instructions', then they may be playing the game of 'showing appreciation for the nurse's time and effort'. Thinking through such ideas helps us to avoid thinking of the patients language as 'lying', 'ignorance' or 'insincerity'.

This raises an important point about the relevance to nursing of philosophical discussion about language. It is not only a discussion which can be applied to nurses' language, but also to patients' language, and even more importantly to interaction between nurse and patient. The discussion so far has concentrated on some of the problems that nurses have encountered with language, but this can suggest that it is a problem internal to nursing, in other words that it concerns mainly the language that they use to themselves. This can be thought of as one type of language game, i.e. the nursing language game, which has a different set of rules to other language games. Take, for example, the often crtiicized use of jargon in nursing. Using abbreviations or slang terms is a form of shorthand which can convey messages quickly to other nurses, and as such needs to follow rules about clarity and brevity. The use of jargon can also, of course, be used in another language game, that of displaying membership of a particular group, in which case the rules are about uniformity. When the language game changes to one about communicating sensitively and clearly to patients, however, jargon is less likely to meet the rules.

Take, for example, a common piece of jargon used in coronary care units – the term 'cabbage' used to talk about coronary artery bypass grafting. The jargon is clearly quicker and simpler than using the full term, and when nurses use it in talk to each other, it presents few problems. If, however, the term is used in conversation with a patient or visitor it can produce disconcerted or distressed responses – being told that the patient in the next bed is 'a cabbage' has a lot of other meanings. If the language game is about giving sympathetic and reassuring information, then 'cabbage' clearly will not do. We might also worry, of course, about what it is that such jargon communicates to the people who use it – does talking about 'cabbages' help nurses to think about patients as human beings or as vegetables?

This is not to suggest that nurses need to explicitly and laboriously enumerate different language games that they might play, with a corresponding set of rules for each; such a course would be fruitless given, as Wittgenstein argued, that rules cannot cover all eventualities. What we do need to do, however, is think about the language game that we are playing and avoid mixing them up. This has implications for much of the research in communication in nursing, which typically attempts to classify communication as being 'therapeutic', 'social' or 'instrumental', for example. When observing nurses talking to patients, such researchers then try to count the frequency of the different types of communication, and/or describe the nature of the language used. Such research seems to be relying implicitly on the idea of the language game of nurse–patient communication as being bound by certain rules, and adherence to these rules is used to classify observations as examples of 'good' or 'bad' interaction. The questions that we must ask about this sort of research, however, are not just about the findings, but whether the researchers have got the right game or not.

More generally, the philosophical discussion of language has relevance for much other nursing research, particularly when it involves talking to patients or nurses. The 'mapping' view of language seems to operate quite strongly here, when interview data are seen to represent inner feelings, and interview technique is discussed in terms of whether it 'really' taps into feelings. Perhaps it might be more useful to think of the interview as a particular sort of language game, and one in which different participants might well have different sorts of rules.

Much of this chapter has been 'playing around with words', debating their nature, significance, use and effect. Endless disputes of this kind tend to provoke the reaction that all we are doing is just playing around with words. But sometimes playing around with words is just what we need to do. Because the words we use structure the way that we think. And we often need to 'play around' with the way we think in order to find new ways of thinking. So, while it is true that some disputes about the concepts of nursing can seem 'semantic', this does not necessarily mean that they are only semantic.

Language is constitutive of our relationships but it is not the only thing that is constitutive of those relationships. The relationships that we have with patients (or clients or customers) are constituted by our (and their) environments, motives, attitudes and beliefs. Language, however, is the main way in which we convey and construct these relationships, and by examining our language we can come to examine these other elements as well. Language is not something that comes from outside us; it is not external to our life. Yet it is not entirely internal either; we do not all have private languages . Language is therefore a social, interactional thing, and as nurses engaged in social, interactional practice, we need to place our disputes and definitions and language use in this context.

References

Foucault, M. 1976: *Birth of the clinic*. London: Tavistock.
Frege, G. 1979: *Posthumous writings*. Oxford: Basil Blackwell.
Monk, R. 1990: *Ludwig Wittgenstein: the duty of genius*. London: Vintage.
Orwell, G. 1962: *1984*. Secker and Warburg.
Von Leibniz, G.W. 1973: *Philosophical writings*. London: Dent, Everyman's Library.
Whorf, B.L. 1956: *Language, thought and reality*. Cambridge, MA: MIT Press.
Wittgenstein, L. 1961: *Tractatus Logico-philosophicus*. London: Routledge.
Wittgenstein, L. 1967: *Philosophical investigations*. Oxford: Blackwell.

Further reading

Adams, P. (ed.) 1972: *Language in thinking*. Harmondsworth: Penguin.

Austin, J.L. 1962: *How to do things with words*. Oxford: Oxford University Press.

Austin, J.L. 1962: *Sense and sensibilia*. Oxford: Oxford University Press.

Ayer, A.J. 1971: *Language, truth and logic*. Harmondsworth: Pelican.

Baudrillard, J. 1988: *Selected writings*. Cambridge: Polity.

Blackburn, S. 1984: *Spreading the word – groundings in the philosophy of language*. Oxford: Clarendon Press.

Chomsky, N. 1975: *Reflections on language*. Glasgow: Fontana.

Derrida, J. 1976: *Writing and difference*. London: Routledge.

Dummet, M. 1973: *Frege – philosophy of language*. London: Duckworth.

Fodor, J.A. 1978: *The language of thought*. Sussex: Harvester Press.

Foucault, M. 1972: *The archaeology of knowledge*. New York: Pantheon.

Francis, H. 1975: *Language in childhood*. London: Elek Books.

Gellner, E. 1959: *Words and things*. Harmondsworth: Penguin.

Hacker, P.M.S. and Baker, G.P. 1980: *Wittgenstein – meaning and understanding*. Oxford: Basil Blackwell.

Hacker, P.M.S. and Baker, G.P. 1985: *Wittgenstein – rules, grammar and necessity*. Oxford: Basil Blackwell.

Hacker, P.M.S. 1972: *Insight and illusion*. Oxford: Oxford University Press.

Hacking, I. 1975: *Why does language matter to philosophy?* Cambridge: Cambridge University Press.

Hallet, G. 1977: *A companion to Wittgenstein's 'Philosophical Investigations'*. Ithaca: Cornell University Press.

Harrison, B. 1973: *Form and content*. Oxford: Basil Blackwell.

Lecercle, J.-J. 1985: *Philosophy through the looking glass*. London: Hutchinson.

Linden, E. 1974: *Apes, men and language*. Harmondsworth: Penguin.

O'Conner, A. 1975: *The correspondence theory of truth*. London: Hutchinson University Library.

Pears, D.F. 1967: *Bertrand Russell and the British tradition in philosophy*. Glasgow: Fontana.

Searle, J.R. 1969: *Speech acts – An essay in the philosophy of language*. Cambridge: Cambridge University Press.

Searle, J.R. (ed.) 1971: *The philosophy of language*. Oxford: Oxford University Press.

Sontag, S. 1978: *Illness as metaphor*. New York: Farrar, Straus and Giroux.

Steiner, G. 1967: *Language and silence*. Harmondsworth: Penguin.

9

Looking at changes in nursing

Introduction

We have seen that one of the roles of philosophy is to give us a place from which to view and review the issues that shape our profession. It provides a place which, if it is not completely neutral (as nowhere is), is at least more impartial than the home territories of the various theoretical factions which inform nursing practice. In this book we have looked at the various areas of philosophy, and tried to show how the debates and ideas here can provide a way of thinking through some of the issues which face nurses. It has, however, been difficult to portion up both nursing and philosophy into discrete debates and issues, given that both disciplines are wide ranging in their concerns and debates. In many chapters, therefore, links can be made with other areas – moral philosophy and philosophy of the mind, for example, both have something useful to contribute to debates on the way we treat people. Dividing up nursing and philosophy into these areas, however, has afforded some idea of the scope and nature of philosophy.

In this final chapter, we attempt something different, in that we discuss a more general nursing issue using a more general philosophical approach. Our reason for doing this is to provide some sort of indication of how nurses can use philosophical approaches without necessarily categorizing a problem as 'belonging to' a particular branch of philosophy (and therefore feeling that they have to read all the philosophy in this branch before they can dare to construct any argument) but can use general philosophical principles of argument and logic to examine issues. We have, therefore, selected a nursing issue which is not only important but extremely complex and apparently intractable, and proceeded to break it down into the various positions held, and the founding premises of these positions. Having done this, we look at the logical implications of these starting points – where they will lead us if we follow them to their conclusions – and identify some of the weaknesses in them. When evaluating the weaknesses (and strengths) of the different positions we can then come to some sort of conclusion.

The issue that we have chosen is, indeed, a very general one, i.e. an examination of the changes that are taking place in nursing approaches to patient care. This can be characterized broadly as a move away from the 'old' model of nursing as a series of tasks carried out in a mechanistic but efficient way, to the 'new' model of nursing which seeks to promote individualized non-routinized, holistic approaches. It must be noted, however, that using the terms 'old' and 'new' does not imply that the latter has replaced the former; indeed, one of the interesting points about this change is its incompleteness – that the two models can exist alongside each other with resulting tensions and conflicts. One particularly important role for philosophy is to offer perspectives on the conflict between two models of nursing that are familiar to most of us in name and all of us in practice. In true philosophical tradition, then, we first set out the terms of the debate, with an examination of the models that we discuss.

'Old' nursing

'Old nursing' is predicated upon the view that nursing is best understood in terms of the characteristic tasks, or *functions*, of nursing practice. This is the model of nursing that has dominated since its origins as a recognized profession and its creation is popularly attributed to Florence Nightingale. The model has various names, often pejorative: 'task-orientated', 'industrial', 'Fordist', 'functional'.

Elements of 'old' nursing

A first philosophical task – one of analysis – is to try and break this model down into its elements. The following list is one way of doing this.

1 An emphasis on the physical aspects of illness.

2 A model of the patient as the object of work.

3 The nurse's relationship to the people who are her patients, as opposed to the patient she helps to cure or manage is regarded as, at best, an optional extra and, at worse, a distraction from the nurse's professional duties. But the general truth is: 'cold hands, warm heart' – emotions are hidden behind efficiency.

4 A distinction between ordinary care, which is motivated by personal connection with the one cared for, and professional care, which is motivated by institutional objectives, which is impartial and concerned with the *real* interests of the patient: objectively defined health goals.

5 A definition of nursing functions which is parasitic upon the characteristic functions of doctors.

6 The success of nursing practice is judged by objective rates of medical success.

7 The emphasis is on results and product.

Views of persons

From this we can take the next analytic step, which is to try and categorize these elements. Which belong together? Under what sorts of headings? There will not be only one way of doing this. But doing it at all is a way of beginning to engage with the underlying issues. One way of organizing these themes is to ask: what persons are involved here and what is being said about them? Obviously the persons mentioned are nurses, doctors and patients.

- Ideas about the nurse
  Elements (3), (4), (5) and (6)
- Ideas about the patient
  Elements (1), (2) and, perhaps, (3)
- Ideas about the doctor
  Element (5).

Distinctions

This classification seems to cover most of the ideas but other things are left out or only rather uncomfortably squeezed into a particular box. For example, element (3) is about both patients and nurses together and not really about either separately. Perhaps a more comprehensive approach would be to classify our original ideas in terms of a set of distinctions. When we do this, we can identify distinctions between the following:

- Objective judgements vs. subjective judgements
  Elements (3), (4) and (6)
- Health vs. illness
  Element (1)
- Process vs. product
  Element (7)
- Real interests vs. apparent interests
  Element (4)
- Nursing functions vs. doctor functions
  Element (5)
- Lay care vs. professional care
  Element (4)
- Physical vs. psychological
  Element (1)
- Physical vs. social
  Element (1)
- Persons as persons vs. persons as patients
  Element (3)
- Activity vs. passivity
  Element (2)

On examining these distinctions, it is apparent that our analysis has forced us to recognize points or concepts that are only implicit in the original material. For example, part of element (4), which is described only in terms of a patient's real interest can be seen to contain an implicit contrast with the notion of apparent interest. We can therefore think about what is not discussed as well as about what is discussed. Using this approach to analysis we can also see that some contrasts seem implausible or confusing. For example, can the physical be contrasted with the psychological in the same way as it can be contrasted with the social?

The point of this process of categorization is that even the use of inadequate categories enables us to find some way to think about the ideas. We might now seek to list these distinctions in order of importance or in order of logical sequence. What follows from what? For example, the distinction between lay care and professional care may be thought to give rise to distinctions between subjective and objective judgements – subjective judgements are associated with lay care and hard objective judgements with professional care. We can now ask whether this distinction is justifiable. Similarly, we can ask about the criteria for determining the contrast between a patient's avowed interests and their real interests.

Arguments against 'old nursing'

At some point, the best way to understand a set of ideas is to ask what kinds of criticism have been or could be made of it. What criticisms were, in fact, made of this model of nursing?

Historically, as this model came to be regarded as both inaccurate in its account of what it is like to be a nurse and as dangerously limiting in its account of the ways in which the profession could develop, objections were developed to the old model which were practical, political and philosophical. At the practical level, it was objected that mass treatment was not as efficient as it pretended. Ward-level health care does not necessarily benefit from economies of scale. Though it might be administratively easier to take the whole ward's temperature at 2.30 a.m., in terms of health outcomes this energy was misdirected. In addition, the reduction of nursing to separable tasks often obscured the connections between aspects of a patient's condition which were critical to health. One nurse administers the drugs and another takes temperatures but who is able to discover the need for antipyretics?

Politically, the objections were complex. The more distant and sporadic the relation of health-care workers to patients, the greater their power and status. Patients were effectively barred from a say in their own medical destiny, as decisions were made by those with whom they had least contact. The implication of this was that many of the decisions affecting patients were taken without consulting them in a meaningful way.

One way in which health organizations tried to institutionalize respect for patient autonomy was to recreate the patient as a client or even a customer. This was ironic. Although the perceived need for greater respect for the patient's own choices seemed to many to be part and parcel of treating the whole person, describing the patient as a 'customer' seemed to reduce them to a sum of essentially economic choices. There was a notion of the patient not as a 'health citizen', but as a 'health consumer' which won the day.

The apparent confluence of industrial and military models seemed, to its opponents, to characterize the old approach. Philosophically, the older model seem committed to outdated and parochial conceptions of persons, of health and of health care. What conception of what a person is could sustain the notion of the patient as a set of medical presentations? What was it that could give a sense to seeing a person as separate from their (ill) body?

This defining feature of the old model could be traced to its Cartesian inheritance. As we saw in Chapter 3, Descartes' account of the nature of mind was designed not so much to save the human soul for theology as to save the body for science. The effect of draining the body of psychological significance was to make it both possible and permissible to think of the body as just another of the complex physical entities to be found in nature. The body could be understood as human machinery and was therefore rendered amenable to scientific investigation. Medical science was by far the most significant beneficiary of this perspective. Medical science, as a science, now seemed to be premised on treating human bodies as psychologically inert. Medicine and mechanism seemed made for each other.

An important claim of feminist philosophers was that Cartesian dualism was not what it seemed. The 'dirty' bodily functions of menstruation and reproduction could be assigned to the body whilst the mind remained unaffected in its lofty purity. Since women were defined in terms of sexual and reproductive function, dualism involved a covert identification of men with intellect and reason and women with physicality and brute instinct. Clarity and certainty lay with the mind; confusion and uncertainty with the body. Cartesianism dressed male domination as metaphysics.

It seemed important to feminists both to reject the covert identification of the mind–body divide with the gender divide and to reject the evaluation of bodily life as inferior to the life of the mind. Some thinkers stressed therefore that an emphasis of the life of the body signified a proper engagement with the world. Men claimed to be involved in the real (because public) world whilst women were confined to the, by contrast, unreal, domestic sphere. In reality, it was women who were involved in the real (because physical) world and men who sought to distance themselves from it.

This feminist critique seems to resonate with disquiet about medicine's conception of the patient. It was men, in the role of doctors, who were charged with the job of repairing or re-engineering the human machine but their intervention was wrapped in scientific gloves and therefore protected from contamination. By contrast, women, in the role of nurses, dealt with the body directly and must therefore already be contaminated.

In addition, however, since doctors are primarily technicians, the role of dealing with the psychological context of illness fell to women as well. The price of a doctor's dealings with bodies was to eschew engagement with the persons those bodies belonged to. Physical intervention is bearable only because the body has become mere matter and therefore not dirty. Whereas the price of nurses' engagement with bodies was to manage the emotional implications of treatment as well as the sordid physical implications. These are the sorts of reflections which led the feminist critique of the old model.

Under this assault from these different perspectives – practical, philosophical and political – the old model came to seem moribund, ridiculous, and even morally outrageous. What, however, was to replace it?

'New' nursing

The opposing model developed by contrast with the old. The new model was to be neither industrial nor military but personal. This model too has enjoyed a diverse set of labels: 'the nursing process', 'patient-centred nursing', 'primary nursing', 'case management' and, more generally, 'humanistic' and 'holistic' care. Early models were developed in the 1950s. But, in the UK at least, it reached its heyday in the 1970s. A milestone here was the recognition of this new 'nursing process' approach by the General Nursing Council in the nursing syllabus of 1977.

The new model now enjoys theoretical dominance in official nursing literature. This is the way that nurses are trained, and the way in which they purport to practice. In reality, of course, the older model retains some influence, and the victory of the new model is far from complete

Elements of 'new' nursing

Characteristics of this model are:

- An emphasis on the patient as person.
- A definition of nursing functions which is independent of the characteristic functions of doctors.
- A thorough-going acknowledgement of the psychological and social contexts of illness.
- An emphasis on health rather than illness.
- Definitions of successful nursing practice in terms of a range of outcomes.
- An emphasis on process, rather than product.
- The nurse's relationship to the people who are his or her patients is regarded as partly constitutive of the nursing role.
- A emphasis on a new role of the nurse as patients' advocate in their relation to health institutions.

Views of persons

Categorizing the elements of new nursing, as before, in terms of what is being said about the roles of nurse, patient and doctor, we can see that in many ways the ideas are very different to old nursing. The nurse is presented as an autonomous practitioner, very much with the patient. The patient is seen as a complex individual with a range of needs. The doctor has become almost invisible.

Distinctions

Returning to the distinctions identified within the old model of nursing, we can see that new nursing has modified many of these. First of all, the new model involves the denial of contrasts which were integral to the older model. For example, it denies the earlier contrast between, on the one hand, physical elements and, on the other, psychological and social elements. Linked to this is a denial of the contrast between the identity of someone as a patient and their identity as a person.

In place of the lost contrasts, the new model introduces some new contrasts. For example, implicit in the idea of the nurse as the patient's advocate are a whole set of new oppositions:

- Patient vs. doctor
- Patient vs. institution
- Nurse vs. institution
- Nurse vs. doctor

Finally, it is significant that this model shares some of the distinctions of the earlier model but puts its emphasis on the other element of the contrast. For example, this model also makes the distinctions:

- Process vs. product
- Nursing functions vs. medical functions
- Health vs. illness
- Care for individuals vs. fairness to individuals as members of groups

But here the process of nursing is emphasized and the importance of the product downgraded. Illness is seen as a concept which is parasitic upon a well-defined concept of health. Finally, the distinction between the characteristic functions of nurses and those of doctors is maintained. What changes is the claim about the relationship between them; what was a parasitic relationship is now seen portrayed as a relationship between equal and independent practitioners.

Objections to 'new' nursing

Having clarified the nature of new nursing in this way, we can now turn, as we did with the old model, to some of the objections which are being made to it. One striking irony of these models is that the functional model of nursing, with its covert acknowledgement of 'cold hands, warm heart', is one largely constructed by patients. Whereas, the humanistic model, which stresses the importance of a personal relationship with real persons is one largely constructed by nurses and nursing theorists.

At least some of the other objections to new nursing arise from the context in which nursing often takes place: a large bureaucratic health service. Individualized care does not always fit in with organizational practices and objectives, and organizations provide services for broadly defined groups of patients rather than precisely assessed individuals. To take just one example, catering; it can be seen that hospital kitchens can only cope with general dietary preferences, and whatever the nurse and patient think is a desirable diet will be modified by the complexities of planning to feed hundreds of patients with limited budgets, staff and resources.

Other problems for new nursing arise from the conflict between the outcome objectives of the organization and the process objectives of holistic care. Outcomes are easier to measure – the length of stay and the mortality rate (although it is more difficult to attribute them to particular causes) – whereas process objectives, about the quality of the patient experience, are less tangible. As organizations become more concerned with measuring performance, the more available measures selected may conflict with new nursing and its criteria for good care.

Alongside these political problems is the issue of professional power and influence. The new model advocates and sometimes assumes that nurses have a degree of control over their practice to an extent that is not enjoyed by nurses generally. The model of nursing developed by Florence Nightingale, where the nurse was directed by the doctor has been enshrined in many health-care systems, with patients being regarded as the responsibility of medical staff, and with all interventions, nursing care among them, being under the control of doctors. With patients 'belonging' to doctors in this way, nurses are often unable to exercise any judgement independently. Patients with the same condition are treated according to the preference of the consultant rather than the nurse, and failure to observe these preferences is treated as incompetence. Pre-operative preparation is one example, where operation sites are prepared according to the surgeons wishes rather than any scientific rationale, and on any one ward patients having the same operation but a different surgeon, may well be subject to a variety of weird and wonderful preparations, regardless of nursing opinion. The adoption of new nursing in these circumstances of medical control is extremely problematic.

Medical and bureaucratic control also extends beyond the details of daily practice to the basic resources needed for the new nursing. Staffing levels and levels of support and training need to be adequate, otherwise individualized care is given sketchily and inefficiently. These are practical objections to new nursing. If these resources are not available, then nurses are driven back to a 'safety-first approach' to care, in which there is a concentration on keeping patients alive, and treating the rest as an optional luxury, to be addressed when there is more time or more staff.

One argument for the new nursing, of course, was that it would help to define the area of nursing expertise and authority, and therefore give nursing a means of arguing for the resources which it feels that it needs, but this has stimulated counterclaims that the new nursing is simply about raising the professional status of nurses. This accusation sees increased autonomy for nurses as a selfish, self-promoting strategy, which has more to do with battles over the patient than for the patient. In seeking to assert the new nursing, on the grounds of improved care, the profession therefore runs the risk of seeming to promote its own interests rather than patients.

This gives rise to dilemmas for nurses who may find it easier to apologize for the new nursing than promote it, but it also reflects some philosophical problems inherent in the assumptions made about new nursing. The assumption made that nurses' and patients' interests are the same rather than conflicting raises questions about the nature of their roles and the relationship between them which are part of a philosophical debate about ethics, rights, duties and politics. There are also questions to be raised about the particular conception of patients' needs that the new nursing promotes, namely that health care should be holistic and humanistic, and how this view is justified. While holistic care, attending to the social and psychological aspects of health as well as the physical may well seem logical, there are questions about its ethical and political basis – at what point does holistic care become intrusive and authoritarian?

The result of these questions for many nurses is a bad professional conscience – 'political correctness' when talking about their work, but actually doing something different. They observe the new theoretical verities when talking about their work, at least in situations where they feel obliged to conform to accepted professional mores. But in practice or informally amongst themselves, the vocabulary of the older model creeps back, and nursing becomes again a matter of getting through the work. Getting on with their work seems to involve renewing loyalties with older models which officially have been discarded. This gives them a hostile view of all theories which come to seem irrelevant to practice.

For some, this is testament to a healthy scepticism about theories which is a necessary virtue for any nurse. However, the contrast is not between theory and practice, but between different kinds of practice arising from different types of theories and values. The danger is that unreflective scepticism about theories becomes an ideology in itself, and stifles critical debate. It is then possible for nurses to become victims of theory without even knowing it.

Reflecting on the 'old' and 'new' models

In reflecting on these models, the first thing to get clear about is the nature of models themselves. It is tempting to think of models as descriptions of things in the world which are true, false, or something in between. The only test is how accurate and how precise their representation is. This is misleading. The point of models is to not to be more or less true, but more or less useful. After all, the perfect map is not the same size and scale as the landscape that it maps.

A particular aspect of nursing models is that they are, appropriately, value-driven. In other words, they are reflections of how people think things ought to be, rather than how they are. For a profession concerned with the care of people, values are inherent in any description of their work that such professionals proffer, but when evaluating these models any objections made can be easily cast by others as uncaring. The models can become slogans, and the debate can degenerate into exchanges of insults rather than a careful examination of the propositions put forward.

In the sections above, we outlined the objections to both models on a philosophical, political and a practical level, and our account found more objections to the old model than to the new. Those made against the new model could conceivably be dismissed as being simply indicative of a particular point in nursing history, when new ideas are in the process of being adopted, and practical and political problems are being sorted out. There are, however, some more enduring philosophical problems with new nursing, which are not simply teething problems. Disentangling and identifying these problems, however, is a difficult process which involves wading through a lot of slogans, rhetoric and shibboleths, so the process of analysis needs to begin with the fundamentals – looking at the basic distinctions that are proposed and identifying any problems with them. It is then possible to go further and look at conflicts between the distinctions, or to begin to examine the types of difference between them.

We saw that the new model differs from the old in different *kinds* of ways. It rejects some distinctions, introduces new distinctions and modifies the distinctions it retains. Recognizing that there are these kinds of difference between the models helps to create an agenda for negotiation between them. It is always difficult to make progress from head-on clashes between different perspectives. But by refining our understanding of the disagreements, breaking it down into different elements, we are more easily able to ask the questions which make agreement and progress possible. Are the rejected distinctions entirely redundant? Or can they have a place in the new model without compromising its new distinctions? Are the new distinctions really tenable? Where there is agreement about the tenability of particular distinctions, can the change in emphasis be regarded as useful and productive only in some circumstances and contexts?

The point of the kind of analysis we have been engaged in then is not to defuse the disagreements in the hope of a cosy accommodation but to more precisely define the character of the disagreements so that the right and relevant ideas and arguments can be deployed, defended and developed. The effect of this process, and it is a characteristic effect of philosophy, is to enable protagonists of these perspectives to open up a kind of gap between themselves and their own ideals. To use a military metaphor, they are no longer mere infantry, defending their positions on the ground, but generals able to see the strategic view of the conflict. This can give both sides the kind of detachment from their own position which far from meaning an abandonment of their commitment to their ideas allows them to manage this commitment more effectively.

When we get the required kind of reflective distance from the two models, we are afforded new perspectives. It may be that the clash between the positions is more complex than we previously thought, demanding more detailed analysis of particular ideas or that it is more simple, perhaps allowing for easier resolution.

We will look at three particular elements in the clash between these models, the differing emphasis on care and justice, the emergence of holistic nursing, and the issue of patient advocacy.

Care or justice?

One of the founding principles (and therefore problems) of new nursing is that it trades on notions of care rather than justice. In other words, the concentration on an individualized approach, with 'caring' as its aim, tends to ignore the philosophical debates which surround the provision of services to a wider population. This is not just a practical or political limitation of new nursing, but it is a philosophical one too. One question that can be asked is whether nurses have a duty to consider health care beyond the individual patient, and to accept that limitations of services to the individual may be necessary to provide wider services to a population. This can be cast as a conflict between utilitarian and deontological ethical principles, but there are also questions to be asked about the way in which nurses are educated and the scope of their practice. For nurses to take on board wider health-care issues, their education needs to equip them to do so, and in this sense, the concentration in the nursing syllabi on individualized care is inadequate.

It is weak because assuming that consideration of the care of individuals can be simply multiplied to apply to populations is a fallacious assumption to make. This is not simply a statistical issue about the generalization from individuals to populations, but is an issue about the qualitative difference between the health-care needs and goals of the two. An individual patient may have specific and well-defined needs in a particular context at a particular time, but a population is altogether more amorphous, diverse and volatile.

If nurses, however, are happy with this focus on individualized care, then they must accept the implications of it, especially that any claims to be part of wider policymaking are made more strongly by other interested groups – politicians, administrators and policy experts. The role of the nurse can, therefore, be to provide a touchstone of concrete examples of the effects of policies, the fine detail of care which the larger picture obscures. This necessary relationship between the broad principles of policy and the minutiae of practice seems to provide the most useful way in which nurses can contribute to debates about justice in health care. Conversely, however, ideas about justice can inform daily practice. As we argued in Chapter 7, many nursing decisions invoke, at some level, considerations about fairness, equity and rights, the problem being that this is not always explicit.

In making the distinction between care and justice, therefore, the new model runs the risk of making justice someone else's concern. What we may conclude is that a corrective to this approach is needed. Managing the boundaries between the broad principles of policy and the minutiae of practice may provide the most useful way in which nurses can make their contribution.

Holism – is it justified? Are people always connected to their illness?

New nursing is predicated on care, but of a particular type and form, holistic care, and this gives rise to a set of problems which are to do with the justification of holistic nursing care, the implications of it, and the conflicts it creates with other nursing values. Put very simply (and probably too crudely for advocates) holistic approaches to care focus on the patient as a whole person, as someone with biological, social and psychological needs, rather than reducing them to an illness. There is some justification for holism, in that many health problems have an impact on the psychological and social functioning of the people who have them, and to ignore these aspects of health is likely to prove, at the very least, inadequate and inefficient.

It is, however, entirely possible for people to experience illness in a reductionist way, that is as a purely physical phenomenon which has little or no effect on their social lives, their self-esteem, or their conception of self. In other words an illness can be experienced by a person as something which happens to them, not as something which is them. By adopting a holistic view, therefore, the nurse may be in danger of at least confusing and at most angering people who do see their health problem as the invasion of a virus, an accident of fate or simply an event in their lives rather than an integral part of themselves. Linking the whole person to an illness, then, can have problematic consequences – it is one thing to say that an illness is part of a person, but quite another to say that a person is part of an illness. By making the first connection we may be saying something useful, but by making the second connection we may be claiming more for holism than it warrants.

A further problem with holistic nursing arises from this point. If we insist on seeing health problems as inextricably linked to all areas of life, then does this give nurses some justification for intervening beyond the immediate health-care arena? If health problems are linked to poverty, poor housing, irresponsible behaviour, or inadequate parenting, then what, exactly, should be the nurse's role in all of this? While some may, and do, argue that nursing should 'address' these issues, the details of how this should be done remain constrained by the statutory role, knowledge and power of the nurse. Furthermore, there is an understandable discomfort at the thought of nurses taking on such a potentially invasive role in people's lives.

Nurses intervening in all areas of people's lives is an idea which is distasteful to many given that it potentially involves an infringement of people's privacy and liberty. Not only is this problematic in itself, but it also creates a paradox within new nursing, which holds dear the ideas of patient empowerment and respect for individual's wishes. Interventions, then, must be wide ranging, to meet the demands of holism, but must not be coercive or intrusive, as this will offend against the principles of empowerment. What is left is a position in which nurses will try to 'educate' people about their lifestyle, but leave the decisions about change to them. This is a difficult line to tread, and one that is further complicated by another element of new nursing – the argument that nurses should act as advocates for patients in order to empower them to direct their health care.

A related problem with new nursing is the way in which it can seem to focus more on the psychosocial aspects of care than the physical: the etheralization of the body. While holistic approaches to care may well have provided a timely correction to mechanistic approaches which centre on the body alone, there is a danger that the body can be forgotten in new nursing. The emphasis on helping the patient to understand their health problem can detract from helping them to recover from it. Again, it is questionable whether patients would share this view of care. For them, it may be a priority to get their body sorted out by experts, much in the same way that someone might take their car to a garage. Like taking a car for repair, patients may not want to know a great deal about how the problem is dealt with, and they may simply want it dealt with quickly and competently, so that they can get on with their lives. The concern may be simply with mechanics.

This possibility of non-holistic models of health care in patients calls into question the justification of holistic models in nurses, especially as these nursing models are predicated upon the assumption that nurses and patients work in partnership, and that their interests and concerns are the same. Imposing holistic models on patients contravenes the principles of partnership and respect for patients, and one way round it is to argue that some patients suffer from a form of 'false consciousness', that their position is based on a lack of awareness. This seems to be a very patronizing position to take, and one not very far from the one traditionally taken by medical staff, that they know best.

To reject new nursing on these grounds, and return to the old nursing, however, would be a premature decision to take, and one that would not necessarily be in the interests of patients. To return to a model where psychological and social aspects of health were ignored, and patients were informed as little as possible, seems to be a retrograde step and to ignore all of the problems with the old nursing that stimulated change. It seems that the question raised by new nursing are different and useful questions to ask, and though they may be difficult, there is at least a genuine concern for the patient which was not entirely apparent in the old model of nursing.

Patient advocacy

This seems to stem from ideas that nurses are more able to understand and present patients' views because of their greater intimacy with them. While this may be the case for some nurses and some patients, it is noteworthy that the new model deals in the contrasts patient vs. doctor, patient vs.

institution, nurse vs. institution and nurse vs. doctor, but it tends to ignore the obvious omission of patient vs. nurse. This omission glosses over the fact that other people may be better equipped to be patient advocates than nurses, and furthermore that there will be conflicts between patients and nurses. It may be the case that some patients will want someone to act as an advocate for them in order to present their view to nurses!

The assumption of common goals which underpins notions of nurses as advocates also glosses over problems of influence and power in the relationship between nurses and patients. Although there is an explicit commitment to empowerment of patients in new nursing, the issue of nurse power is less openly discussed. Part of empowering patients involves providing them with the information necessary for them to make choices about their care. Given, however, that nurses have a degree of knowledge and experience which is not enjoyed by many patients, the information that they provide must be necessarily condensed and simplified. In this process of simplification, there is the danger of bias, that the complexities of the decision can be presented in such a stark way that the patient's conclusion can be directed by the nurse. Conversely, in an attempt to be even-handed, the nurse can provide information which is cloaked in uncertainty and qualification to such an extent that the patient is unable to decide between options.

At this point the nurse is in danger of looking as if she cannot decide herself and claims to have some sort of expertise become questionable. As the patient expects some degree of knowledge, competence or expertise from those caring from them, this calls the basis of the relationship into question. Empowering patients then, cannot mean giving them all the information that the nurse has. Most people will not have this amount of time. However, selectively condensing information is also problematic.

The debate also has to be set in the context of wider social change. It is not simply internal to nursing. As naive acceptance of all experts diminishes, and psychological language enters everyday conversation, nursing has to change to reflect this. This is not only because patients are members of a changing society, but because nurses are too.

Conclusion

Despite the issues and problems that we have identified with new nursing, it seems to be a more positive line to take than simply staying with the old model. The issues raised by new nursing are certainly more interesting than those raised by task-allocation models, where the only questions were about how quickly and efficiently care could be delivered. That the new nursing throws into sharp relief questions about differences between nurses and patients seems to be potentially more productive than a situation where these differences were dismissed as unimportant or non-existent, and at least the new nursing provides some sort of space for these questions to be debated. Without this debate, however, new nursing becomes just another set of rules which can be misinterpreted and misused.

To return to the point that we made earlier, models are not descriptions but instruments for thinking. It is mistaken to talk about them as true or false. We should therefore ask whether they are useful or not. By this criterion, we can conclude that new nursing is useful, given that it has stimulated a range of questions which are fundamental rather than superficial to health care. Questions about patients' ideas on health, the imbalances of knowledge and, therefore, power between nurses and patients, the limits and boundaries of nursing care, and the rights of patients, seem to be very useful questions to ask. They may not be answered definitively, and any answers offered may stimulate further questions, but the importance of debate lies in the process, not the product. If new nursing leads nurses to challenge their assumptions and practice, then it will have served some purpose.

In order to conduct these debates, however, nursing needs to stand outside ideology and eschew the sloganeering endemic in ideological conflicts. Here we can use philosophy where everything is up for grabs, assumptions challenged and arguments examined critically. Philosophy is an activity rather than a set of doctrines, which may disconcert those who like their ideas cut and dried rather than provisional and temporary. It is, however, a very public activity, where ideas are laid out and examined, and this is something which nurses have traditionally been wary of. As an occupation, we have perhaps been more concerned with presenting a united front to the world, and are uncomfortable with the idea of acrimonious disputes which can divide us to no great benefit. We have to accept, however, that nursing, working as it does in many different contexts, with many different people, and with many different goals, cannot be entirely uniform in its ideas, and philosophy offers one way of exploring this diversity.

References

General Nursing Council of England and Wales. 1977: *Training syllabus. Register of nurses. General nursing*. London: General Nursing Council for England and Wales.

Further reading

Lawler, J. 1991: *Behind the screens: nursing, somology and the problem of the body.* Edinburgh: Churchill Livingstone.
Smith, P. 1992: *The emotional labour of nursing.* London: Macmillan.

Index